Depression & Your Thyroid

What You Need to Know

GARY S. ROSS, MD

PETER J. BIELING, PH.D.

New Harbinger Publications, Inc.

Distributed in Canada by Raincoast Books.

The Thyroid Gland illustration is used with permission from the University of Michigan Health System, September 2005.

Cover design by Amy Shoup; Acquired by Jesse O'Brien; Edited by Kayla Sussell; Text design by Tracy Marie Carlson

Library of Congress Cataloging-in-Publication Data

Ross, Gary.
   Depression and your thyroid : what you need to know / Gary Ross and Peter J. Bieling.
         p. cm.
   Includes bibliographical references.
   ISBN 1-57224-406-2
   1. Thyroid gland—Diseases—Popular works. 2. Thyroid gland—Diseases—Complications—Popular works. 3. Depression, Mental—Popular works. I. Bieling, Peter J. II. Title.
   RC655.R68 2006
   616.4'4—dc22

                                                            2005035664

New Harbinger Publications' Web site address: www.newharbinger.com

08   07   06
10   9   8   7   6   5   4   3   2   1
First printing

To my patients who, for thirty years,
it has been my honor to serve.

—Dr. Gary Ross

For Audrey

—P.J.B.

Contents

Acknowledgments

I wish to express my gratitude to the following people who helped contribute to this book. Many thanks to David Grant for proofreading so carefully and locating all the references that were needed. Kayla Sussell at New Harbinger was an invaluable editor who helped us craft the writing and gave such valuable feedback as the book came together. Thanks also to my wife, Karen, for her love and support during this project and to friends and family who helped me out with my "distraction coping."

—P.J.B.

My thanks to Dr. Matt McKay, Kayla Sussell, Jess O'Brien, and Heather Mitchener at New Harbinger Publications. Thank you to the following people for the work they have done and continue to do: Dr. Tapan Audhya at Vitamin Diagnostics for our discussions on thyroid testing; Patricia Puglio, Executive Director of Broda O. Barnes Research Foundation for our discussions over the years; Dr. Peter Singer and Dr. John Nicoloff from Keck School of Medicine at the University of Southern California; Dr. David Quig at Doctors Data Laboratory; Dr. Richard Lord at Metametrix Clinical Laboratory; Dr. Aristo Vojdani at Immunosciences Laboratory; Dr. Omar Amin at Parasitology Center; Dr. Kamal Henin at Diagnos-Techs; Dr. Corene Humphreys at Great Smokies Laboratory; Dr. Nick Harris at IGeneX Lab; David Berg and Dr. Harold Harrison at Hemex Lab; Dr. Gottfried

Kellermann at Neurosciences Laboratory; Dr. Jeff Young at Hunter Laboratory; Dr. James Fitzwater at Quest Laboratory; Dr. Steve Harris; Dr. Patricia Kane; Dr. Carl Mani of Diagnostic Radiologists of San Francisco; Dr. Russell Jaffe of Elisa Act Laboratory; Dr. Jonathan Wright; Dr. Alan Gaby; and Dr. Michael Gerber. Thank you to the pharmacists at Women's International Pharmacy, especially Kathy, Tammy, Cathy, Sue, and Chris; the pharmacy staffs at Belmar Pharmacy; Wellness Pharmacy; College Pharmacy; Apothecure; Key Pharmacy; and Bellevue Pharmacy. Thank you to Tom Strange, Pattie MacDonald, Tracy Williams, and Peter Caron. Thank you to my wife, Kathleen, for her enthusiasm and support and for sharing my interest in the pursuit and understanding of true health.

—Dr. Gary Ross

Introduction

IS THIS BOOK FOR YOU?

Let's suppose that once upon a time you suspected you had a low thyroid. Whether you realized it was a part of your family's medical history or you read something about a possible connection between depression and thyroid, you asked your doctor to test your thyroid. If your doctor ordered laboratory testing for your thyroid function, the chances are good that you were told that the tests were returned "in the normal range."

The questions is this: "normal" according to what criteria and which tests?

Not so happily ever after, along with the information that your thyroid was fine, you may have continued to experience worsening symptoms. The information may not have been entirely correct. It is our hope that this book will provide you with the understanding you need to become an empowered patient. Such patients help their doctors in improving the quality of their lives. Knowing the right questions to ask is almost as important as obtaining the correct answers.

WHO THE AUTHORS ARE

Chapters 1 through 7 were written by Dr. Gary Ross. In his private clinical practice, Dr. Ross has successfully treated hundreds of patients suffering from depression caused by low thyroid. He knows firsthand how a badly functioning thyroid can damage the quality of your life. His professional experience makes him uniquely qualified to inform you about all of the medical aspects of the problem and, more importantly, what to do about such medical issues. Here's what he has to say about the thyroid gland and depression.

"I wish I had counted all the times patients have reported to me that they had been informed that their thyroid test results were normal; at the same time, they also reported experiencing most if not all of the symptoms of correctable hypothyroidism. Regrettably, this scenario happens repeatedly in my practice. The importance of correcting a low thyroid condition cannot be overstated. Without exaggeration, it is safe to say that a low thyroid condition can be the crucial difference between leading a life of miserable, helpless suffering or a normal life. In *Depression and the Thyroid: What You Need To Know*, you will gain a deeper understanding of hypothyroidism and its many signs and symptoms. You will learn how to determine if hypothyroidism is at the root of your depression.

"For a solid understanding of the process toward thyroid health, I begin our book with a discussion about the thyroid gland itself. Then the thyroid hormones and their function are discussed, and there is talk about the T3 and T4 and thyroid receptors. I will go into the checklist of hypothyroid symptoms and tell you where and how to obtain proper laboratory testing. I will go into the treatment possibilities, including completely natural supplements, and I will also address certain dietary changes that work for some people."

Chapters 8 through 12 were written by Dr. Peter Bieling. Dr. Bieling, like Dr. Ross, is extremely well-qualified to address these issues. A clinical psychologist, he is currently employed as the manager of Mood, Anxiety, and Women's Health Concerns at St. Joseph's Hospital in Ontario, Canada.

In the second part of the book, Dr. Bieling offers psychological strategies to overcome the depression that can result from a thyroid condition. His chapters offer a variety of strategies for creating a healthy balance in your life, reducing stress, designing positive reinforcement plans, and exploring the ways that your relationships may be contributing to your condition. Here's what Dr. Bieling has to say about depression.

"Because depressed people often have patterns of negative thinking that cause them to go around and around in spirals of negativity making it hard for them to appreciate those aspects of their lives that are going well, I discuss a specific approach called cognitive behavioral therapy (CBT). This form of therapy has proved to be just as effective for treating depression as antidepressant medications are. CBT focuses on the ways that depressed people think, but more than that, on the way they view themselves and their worlds.

"Furthermore, because stress is a known risk factor for getting and staying depressed, I examine some of the ways in which stress is defined, as well as the effects of what stress does to your mind and body. More importantly, I have some valuable suggestions for you on what you can do about the stress in your life.

"Finally, I take a look at relationships, which are often the unintended victims of depression. Although most of us tend to think of depression as a deeply personal illness, that is, as something that happens inside our own minds and bodies, the fallout our relationships experience because of depression is not only very real, it can be very costly. For these reasons I explore some of the common ways that depression undermines healthy and supportive relationships and describe some strategies to minimize the impact of depression on relationships."

WORKING WITH THIS BOOK: KEEP A JOURNAL

There are a number of interactive exercises provided for you in the second half of the book. For that reason it is highly recommended that you buy a blank journal to do the exercises, and to keep a record of your progress. We will both help you to address the specifics of your individual profile and give you the directions you need to work on both the medical and the psychological aspects of a poorly functioning thyroid. Finally, we will refer you to the right organizations to turn to for more information. Read along step-by-step and you'll gain what you need to conquer and demystify a thyroid condition.

Both Dr. Ross and Dr. Bieling hope that their joint efforts to demystify the relationship between thyroid function and depression will be of use to you and help you get started on the path to better health and deeper happiness. Today, given all of the advancements in knowledge about the link between the thyroid and depression, there is no reason anyone should have to deal with depression because of a poorly functioning thyroid. In this book, you will find that help is available. We hope that you will choose to accept it and thus change your life for the better.

CHAPTER 1

Introduction to Hypothyroidism

If you or someone you love suffers from depression, you know how all-encompassing it can be in terms of the overall quality of life. Depression affects every aspect of a person's life. Unlike other disabilities, depression not only alters everything from personal relationships to work abilities, in some cases it also makes it impossible to conduct even the routine tasks of daily life. Then, to make matters even worse, society expects the depressed person to snap out of it, get over it, and get going. Even for those with mild depression who may not even have identified depression as a problem, the mood swings, sluggish thinking, and sleep-pattern disruptions can take a heavy toll.

THE LINK BETWEEN HYPOTHYROIDISM AND DEPRESSION

Fortunately for those in whom depression and hypothyroidism coexist, a profound link has been established between the two states. The reason for calling this linkage "fortunate" is that hypothyroidism is relatively easy to treat and, consequently, so is the depression that results from it. *Hypothyroidism* is the name given to the condition in which the body does not get enough thyroid hormone for optimal brain and body functioning. Note that in this book, the terms "low thyroid" and "hypothyroid" are used interchangeably.

Low thyroid can be an overlooked, undiagnosed cause of depression. We know that people may suffer for years from depression, moodiness, and sluggish thinking either because their thyroid function is never taken into account or because their standardized thyroid tests are returned as "normal." For countless people, an underlying hypothyroid condition remains undiagnosed, untreated, life-limiting, and disabling, often becoming the springboard for further illness. According to Haggerty et al. (1993), patients with subclinical hypothyroidism are reported to have a lifetime prevalence of depression of 56 percent compared to a prevalence of 20 percent among depressed patients who do not have hypothyroidism.

Until recently, there has been a strict reliance on certain basic blood tests and clinical criteria to evaluate the functioning of the thyroid. However, these tests and criteria do not always demonstrate the whole picture of the body's need for thyroid. Although it's true that not all patients with depression are hypothyroid and not all patients diagnosed as hypothyroid are depressed, it has become apparent that properly diagnosing and treating low thyroid can dramatically change a patient's life for the better.

Overt and Subclinical Hypothyroidism

Hypothyroidism includes both overt hypothyroidism which is the most obvious and can be diagnosed with lab testing (see chapter 6) and subclinical hypothyroidism, which is more difficult to diagnosis because some of the laboratory tests appear normal, if only at the low end of normal. In the overt type of hypothyroidism, the lab results are clearly out of range. Lab testing is reported as normal or reported as "out of range" based on a range of normal scale. This scale is determined from 95 percent of the population. Any lab result falling in this range of normal is reported as normal. Any lab result that appears below or above the range of normal on the lab test results is considered out of range.

Subclinical hypothyroidism is a milder form of low thyroid with many of the same symptoms as overt hypothyroidism. As a result of the difficulty in diagnosing it, however, many cases of borderline low thyroid or subclinical hypothyroidism are missed.

The prevalence of overt hypothyroidism, according to Hendrick, Altshuler, and Whybrow (1998), is approximately 2 percent for women and less than 1 percent for men. Subclinical hypothyroidism is also more prevalent among women, occurring in approximately 7.5 percent of women compared to only 3 percent of men. Elderly women have up to a 16 percent rate of subclinical hypothyroidism. Approximately 5 to 15 percent of patients with subclinical hypothyroidism do worsen to develop overt hypothyroidism every year, according to Wiersinga (1995). In my experience, the true incidence of subclinical hypothyroidism is much higher than these figures indicate and accurate diagnosis depends on the types of tests done, the accuracy of those tests, and the interpretation of the laboratory results.

HOW DO YOU KNOW IF YOU HAVE A LOW THYROID?

How would you suspect you have a low thyroid? Each patient is an individual with his or her own presentation of signs and symptoms. Look at the list of signs and symptoms below and compare that list with your own personal set of symptoms. This will allow you to see whether your symptoms match those for hypothyroidism. It's not necessary to match every symptom on the list. Some people with hypothyroidism may experience only two or three symptoms predominantly.

The Signs and Symptoms That May Indicate Hypothyroidism

- Constant fatigue or feelings of exhaustion

- Puffiness of the face

- Trouble getting started in the morning

- Low body temperature

- Sensitivity to cold weather

- Tendency toward cold hands and feet

- Numbness or tingling in arms and legs

- Benign breast lumps

- Tendency toward ovarian cysts and uterine fibroids

- Menstrual irregularity

- Depression

- Introverted, shy, antisocial behavior

- Poor memory or concentration

- Sluggish thinking or thought processes

- Dry skin

- Dry bumps on skin of upper arms and upper legs

- Hair loss

- Loss of hair from eyebrows

- Weak fingernails that peel and crack easily

- Sensation of lack of air supply, or difficulty breathing in or out

- Sluggish reflexes on physical examination

- Unexplained weight gain or difficulty losing weight despite efforts at dieting

- Low blood pressure and slow pulse

- Infertility, repeated miscarriages

- Recurrent infections, including fungal infections

- Low sex drive

Case Histories

Now, let's take a look at some case histories of people who've had low thyroid.

■ Sandra's Story

Sandra was a thirty-year-old woman who was healthy and fit most of her life. She had no trouble juggling her commitments to work, family, friends, and regular exercise, which in her case was jogging. By following her routines she was able to maintain a healthy weight and she had sufficient energy to meet all of her needs.

But after going through a period of extreme stress at her job, Sandra found that she was always exhausted by the end of a normal workday. She also noticed that her thinking seemed sluggish, and she was in a constantly depressed mood. To make matters even worse, she was gaining weight and didn't know why. So, she visited her doctor and a series of tests were done. When her tests results were returned to her doctor, they were all within normal ranges.

Because Sandra's clinical signs and symptoms and her test results didn't meet the classic criteria for diagnosing low thyroid (hypothyroidism), she was told she was basically okay and instructed to take blood tests again in a year. According to her doctor, other factors were to blame for her symptoms. The doctor told her, "Your weight gain is the result of eating too many sweets and carbohydrates and you haven't been exercising enough."

Sandra's experience is fairly common. Often no treatment is offered at all. Period. Patients with low thyroid frequently complain that no matter how little they eat or how often or intensely they work out, their extra weight just stays there without budging. If you are like Sandra, it's likely that you'll be told by your doctor to try antidepressants and to get to the gym more often. There may be some truth to the advice about eating fewer sweets and refined carbohydrates, but the key issue—the status of the thyroid—must be addressed to be corrected.

■ Richard's Story

Richard felt tired his whole life long; even as a child he never seemed to have enough energy for normal living. He had no social life. Because of various stresses and other factors during the course of his life, he gradually became worse as he reached adulthood. He was prescribed thyroid medication as a teenager but he has since discontinued using it. He was told he no longer needed it, because his lab results came back as "normal."

He was so depressed all the time that he had tried a variety of antidepressants like Prozac, Effexor, and Wellbutrin. His doctor continued to prescribe new antidepressants fairly regularly, so Richard spent years trying out new antidepressants or combinations of antidepressants rather than looking for the root of his problem.

As you'll see in chapter 5, antidepressants do have their place in the treatment of depression. However, getting to the root of a thyroid diagnosis can be the difference between feeling barely "okay" and feeling as though you can not only reach your goals, you even have a lot of available energy to use for those pursuits.

In a 1997 article by Henley and Koehnle, twelve studies on depression were cited that demonstrated T3 thyroid hormone treatment is effective as an add-on therapy in approximately 50 to 60 percent of treatment-resistant cases. This is definitely good news for people everywhere who suffer from depression.

T3 (triiodothyronine) is one of the two main thyroid hormones in the blood. It is called T3 because it has three iodine molecules. It is considered to be the active form of thyroid hormone that actually reaches the cells of the body and causes them to function. Supplemental T3 as thyroid replacement therapy is available as a tablet or capsule from different pharmacies.

T4 (tetraiodothyronine) is the other main thyroid hormone. It has 4 iodine molecules and loses one iodine molecule to become T3.

■ Marcia's Story

When Marcia was twenty-one years old, she was placed on thyroid hormone replacement therapy (Armour thyroid). It was determined that she needed it because of a blood test result that showed low levels of T3 and T4. She was kept on Armour thyroid for seven years at the same dosage that was prescribed initially, without ever revisiting the diagnosis or the treatment protocol. She told her doctor that the medication never seemed to make her feel better. She never noticed any improvement in her symptoms, which were lack of energy, dry skin, and depression.

Because no one ever explained the subtleties of hypothyroidism and thyroid replacement to Marcia or showed her all the treatment options that are available, she reached the conclusion that it was just her fate to never feel as energetic as everyone else she knew. However, in spite of her constant low-grade depression, she continued searching for the "real" cause of her difficulties. Clearly, Marcia needed thyroid replacement therapy but she was not receiving the correct amount or type for her body. Marcia's story demonstrates the need to thoroughly test and fine-tune the correct type and dose of thyroid treatment.

These three case histories demonstrate how commonly low thyroid conditions go undiagnosed and untreated and how suboptimally those conditions are treated in most patients. Eventually, these three people all heard something on the radio, or read something in a magazine, that sparked a recognition of their problems and gave them some hope for change. Armed with just a little bit of information about their conditions, they searched for and found knowledgeable health practitioners to treat their subclinical thyroid problems. They were given validation, direction, and hope that their conditions were treatable. After receiving proper treatment for some time they all reported feeling as though they had been given a new lease on life.

THE CORRECT THYROID SUPPLEMENT AND DOSAGE CAN MAKE A HUGE DIFFERENCE

A new patient came to see Dr. Ross after years of having taken the same low dose of Synthroid (a commonly prescribed synthetic form of the thyroid hormone T4) daily. After T3 was prescribed for her (it was added in to her current prescription of Synthroid), the effect within two days was astounding. She called to thank Dr. Ross, saying, "The T3 has made a huge difference. Now, I feel like I'm in the world instead of looking at it." The addition of a low dose of T3 was the sole change made to her medication. (See chapter 7 for a detailed discussion about the treatment of low thyroid with supplementations of T3 and T4 medication.)

When proper clinical analysis and testing have been done and it has been determined that the patient has a low thyroid condition, a slightly drawn-out process may be ahead because the correct type of thyroid replacement therapy and dosages must be continually fine-tuned. It can be exciting for the patient and the knowledgeable physician alike to realize that, in fact, a correctable problem—low thyroid—does indeed exist and that now it is simply a matter of determining a treatment plan.

The patient may have to maintain a degree of patience while chronic symptoms lessen and disappear. Other aspects of the patient's individual treatments may also need adjusting as the patient becomes a more thriving version of him- or herself. As a rule, most patients do not become instantly happy, but their depression does ease up and eventually disappear as they also work on their psychological issues.

The Right Recipe

Finding the correct dosage is a bit like making a soup; you have to add the right amount and perhaps the right combination of thyroid medication to achieve optimal results. This is very important. Frequently, patients will say to their doctors, "But I'm already on thyroid medicine." But, based on treating more than a thousand patients with varying degrees of hypothyroidism, I can tell you that it is worth the time, effort, and expense to find the correct dosage and combination of thyroid medication if the more advanced, specific, and accurate laboratory tests indicate the necessity. (See chapter 6 for details on specific lab testing.)

Once we've diagnosed a specific need for thyroid medication and begun a patient on thyroid hormone replacement of the right type for that person, the beneficial effect can sometimes be observed immediately, even after only one day. It's as if patients snap back to being more like the person they remember themselves as being.

Unfortunately, treatment is not always so dramatic. Sometimes, it can take weeks or months of adjusting and fine-tuning to arrive at the perfect dosage. Unless the doctor and the patient understand that it can be a lengthy process to reach optimal functioning, progress may seem stalled. Nevertheless, with the understanding that finding the correct dosage can be a lengthy process that can require time, effort, and repeat testing, you may experience a remarkable improvement, even a transformation.

Summary

Low thyroid is one of the main frequently overlooked and undiagnosed causes of depression. The status of the thyroid gland is often the key issue in depression and it needs to be addressed and corrected. In most cases, treating low thyroid can improve a patient's depression. It is important to test correctly and to find the right dose and combination of thyroid modalities for success. There are common signs and symptoms that indicate a hypothyroid condition.

CHAPTER 2

Thyroid Basics

THE THYROID GLAND

The *thyroid gland* is a small butterfly-shaped gland located in the front of the neck. It is located below the Adam's apple and the cricoid cartilage and is connected to the trachea by *fascia* (a type of connective tissue). It wraps around the trachea (the windpipe) on both sides. It has two lobes that extend to each side and an isthmus (a narrow part connecting the two lobes) in the middle that gives it its butterfly shape. (See figure 1.1.)

Examining the Thyroid

Normally, in its healthy state, you cannot easily see or feel the thyroid gland in the front of the neck. When the gland is examined by a physician during a physical examination, it is carefully palpated, usually from the front of the neck. When the patient is instructed to swallow, both lobes, one on each side of the isthmus, can be felt by the examining physician as very soft tissues that move up and down slightly. Sometimes, the patient is asked to swallow a few sips of water to help the thyroid gland move up and down with the movement of the trachea. As a rule, the physician does not perform this examination unless the thyroid is obviously enlarged or the patient has complained of a sensation in that area, such as difficulty swallowing.

Thyroid Gland

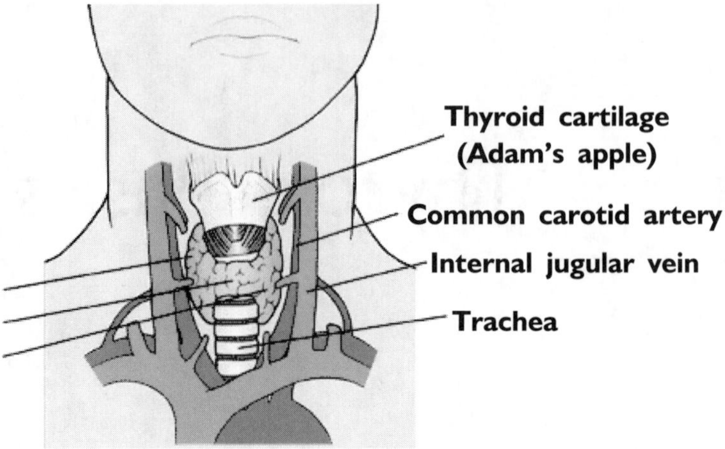

Thyroid cartilage
(Adam's apple)

Common carotid artery

Internal jugular vein

Right lobe

Isthmus

Trachea

Left lobe

Front View

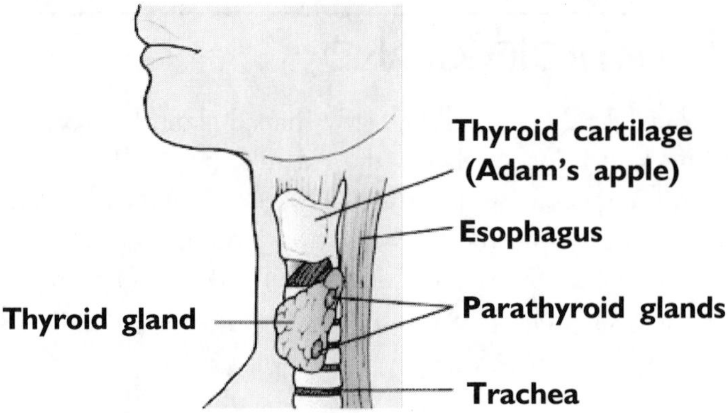

Thyroid cartilage
(Adam's apple)

Esophagus

Parathyroid glands

Thyroid gland

Trachea

Side View

Figure 1.1: The thyroid gland at a glance.

WHAT DOES THE THYROID GLAND DO?

The main purpose of the thyroid gland is to gather up iodine and use it to produce thyroid hormones, which are necessary for metabolism and good mental and emotional functioning. The iodine is taken in through the diet from fish or seaweeds, sea salt, or supplements such as kelp and dulse (sea vegetables). The gland takes up the iodine as iodide (Larsen et al. 2003) and attaches it to a glycoprotein (a combination of protein and carbohydrate) structure called thyroglobulin, adding more iodine molecules.

The Production of T1, T2, T3, and T4 Thyroid Hormones

In the way described above, the thyroid gland produces the individual thyroid hormones T1 and T2 and combines them to form two other thyroid hormones, T3 (triiodothyronine) and T4 (tetraiodothyronine). It starts by adding one iodine molecule to the thyroglobulin, which produces T1. Then it adds another iodine molecule to the thyroglobulin, producing T2. Next, T1 and T2 are combined together to produce T3 and T4. That's it. A total of four of these thyroid hormones is made.

The thyroglobulin itself is made from an amino acid called *tyrosine*. Tyrosine is commonly know for its antidepressant effect. Part of that effect is directly on the brain, affecting the production of some neurotransmitters, but tyrosine also acts to increase the production of thyroid hormones because it is the building block of thyroglobulin. The building blocks for making thyroid hormones include tyrosine, iodine, and *adaptogenic* herbs. Adaptogenic herbs such ginseng, ashwagandha, and rhodiola are believed to have a balancing and stress-reducing effect on the body. They help the body to adapt to stress. (By the way, adaptogenic herbs are also added to these formulas to support the adrenal gland since adrenal support also supports thyroid function, as is discussed in chapter 6.)

Some people take tyrosine tablets or capsules as a nutritional supplement, but the purpose of mentioning tyrosine here is to look at the whole picture of thyroid and depression in order to get to the root of your individual needs. Chapter 7, which is about treatment modalities, discusses tyrosine and other natural supplements that might become a part of your overall treatment picture. Just as the thyroid hormones are continually built step-by-step, we want to consider and understand the thyroid gland's function as it relates to depression step-by-step. We want to see you develop an effective and thorough plan based on proper diagnosis and specific treatment as indicated for you as a specific individual.

The Focus Is on T3 and T4

The focus is on T3 and T4 because among the four thyroid hormones, these are the most important. T1 and T2 are considered to be *precursor hormones.* Precursor hormones are the first steps in building the final end products, T3 and T4. T1 and T2 are the intermediary steps between the thyroglobulin starting material and the final products, the T3 and T4 thyroid hormones.

At any one moment in time, the thyroid gland will contain iodine, thyroglobulin, T1, T2, T3, and T4. There is some information about the function of T2 in the medical literature; however, in the hundreds of articles and studies about thyroid hormones and thyroid function in that literature, the emphasis is on the main thyroid hormones, T3 and T4 (Hendrick, Altshuler, and Whybrow 1998).

Currently, there is very little information available on T1 and T2. In the future, as interest and research into the range of thyroid function in all areas of health expand, we are likely to see more focus on T2. In the meantime, though, in the literature and in everyday clinical practice, T3 and T4 are the thyroid hormones we work with to improve body function, including examining, as we are doing here, the treatment of depression. This doesn't mean that T1 and T2 are excluded from treatment options as they are natural components of the thyroid gland. For example, the thyroid medications Armour thyroid, Westhroid thyroid, and Nature-throid all include T1 and T2 along with T3 and T4 in their preparation.

THE THYROID HORMONES ARE NECESSARY FOR LIFE

The thyroid hormones are necessary for life. The thyroid hormones in the thyroid gland make normal functioning of the metabolism possible.

Normal Functioning Metabolism

Metabolism is the term used to describe the various physical and chemical processes of the body by which the building blocks are produced and eliminated, and by which energy is produced. Metabolism includes the process of building up the thyroid hormones from the thyroglobulin, but it also includes the eventual elimination of the thyroid hormones from the body. This is part of the normal process. The thyroid hormones are always being created and broken down, created and broken down, created and broken down. This is the normal cycle. When this cycle is either interrupted or the thyroid hormones are not adequately produced, problems with metabolism and, of course, thyroid function and other significant health problems such as depression result.

Your metabolism controls the warmth of your body and the energy your body produces. You may be familiar with the concept of a fast metabolism and a slow metabolism. People with a low thyroid definitely have a slower metabolism. Their bodies slow down and become sluggish on many levels. Someone with a slow metabolism may even speak more slowly than someone whose metabolism is normal or fast. When the body moves more slowly, it lacks fire power to burn fat, think fast, stay warm, and excrete waste products. Take another look at the bullet, list of signs and symptoms that may indicate hypothyroidism in chapter 1. All of those seemingly unconnected symptoms are the result of the same problem, an underactive thyroid.

If the metabolism is slow, there is a tendency toward depression. People with slow metabolism might not even think of themselves as being depressed, but they will admit that they lack enthusiasm. With a slow metabolism, sometimes there is a subtle decrease in energy for all of the activities of life. As the thyroid is treated, the metabolism picks up and the symptoms gradually dissipate, including the symptoms of depression. It is our hope that so, too, your understanding of how this all works together will continue to come together.

Now, let's take a look at the different profiles of someone with a normal, good metabolism and someone with a slow metabolism.

CHARACTERISTICS OF A GOOD METABOLISM

The following bulleted items are all indicative of a well-functioning metabolism:

- An excellent body weight in terms of the person's height, bone structure, and age.

- Adequate to abundant energy to get through each day's tasks.

- Consistent energy throughout the day, that is, energy levels don't undergo extreme changes, rising and falling throughout the day.

- Someone with a good metabolism is drawn to eat a healthy diet, balanced with complex carbohydrates such as vegetables and proteins, and experiences limited cravings.

- Healthy skin, hair, and nails.

- Regular bowel movements.

- In women, there is no tendency toward breast lumps, ovarian cysts, uterine fibroids, menstrual irregularities, or infertility.

- Mentally, a good metabolism encourages an optimistic, socially outgoing, conversational personality.

- People with good metabolism have minds that work quickly.

- A good metabolism supports agility and athleticism.

- A good metabolism ensures the absence of muscle cramps.

- A good metabolism supports a "can-do" attitude.

- People with good metabolism tend to run a generally normal temperature.

- People with good metabolism make new connections easily, start new projects with enthusiasm, and have temperaments characterized by hopefulness.

CHARACTERISTICS OF A SLOW METABOLISM

The following bulleted items are all indicative of a poorly functioning metabolism:

- Cold extremities, that is, people with slow metabolism always have cold hands and feet.

- People with slow metabolism are very sensitive to cold; they get very cold too easily, especially in colder weather.

- A slow metabolism tends to build up waste products, and creates difficulty in eliminating waste products.

- People with slow metabolism gain weight rapidly regardless of how much or how little food they consume.

- People with slow metabolism suffer from constipation.

- A slow metabolism causes hair to become dry and coarse.

- A slow metabolism causes skin to be dry and rough.

- In women, a slow metabolism creates a tendency toward breast and ovarian cysts, uterine fibroids, menstrual irregularities, and infertility.

- People with slow metabolism experience many cravings for sugary carbohydrates.

- A slow metabolism provides too little energy to accomplish a day's tasks.

- People with slow metabolism tend to be clumsy and not athletically inclined.

- A slow metabolism creates a tendency toward recurrent muscle cramps.

- People with slow metabolism tend to be mentally slow or dull-witted.

- People with slow metabolism tend to have cognitive difficulties (trouble processing information).

- A slow metabolism is believed to be involved in subtle degrees of ADD (attention deficit disorder).

- A slow metabolism can be involved in subtle depression or major depression.

- People with slow metabolism tend to suffer from continual fatigue; they are always tired, even after a good night's sleep.

- People with slow metabolism lack the energy needed for "staying power"; they tend to lose steam, especially in the afternoon or early evening.

- For people with slow metabolism, life is a constant struggle.

- People with slow metabolism lack the energy to make new connections or start new projects.

- A slow metabolism can create a constant feeling of hopelessness.

The thyroid hormones are considered to be the primary factors affecting metabolism. Additional factors that affect metabolism include other healthy organs, for example, the adrenals and kidneys. However, it is mainly the function of the thyroid gland to regulate metabolism. If anything decreases the production or availability of the thyroid hormones for the cells of the body, it will lower the metabolism, which means you will be more prone toward depression along with many of the other symptoms we've discussed.

Summary

The thyroid gland is located in the front of the neck. Its main function is to produce thyroid hormones. Thyroglobulin is the material from which T1, T2, T3, and T4 (the thyroid hormones) are made. Thyroid hormones are necessary for a well-functioning metabolism and thus for good mental and emotional functioning. The focus is on the T3 and T4 thyroid hormones. People with a low functioning thyroid have a slow metabolism. People with slow metabolisms tend to be depressed.

CHAPTER 3

Vitality and the Thyroid Hormones

THE MANUFACTURE OF THE THYROID HORMONES

As explained in chapter 2, the iodine that is obtained from the diet attaches to thyroglobulin in the thyroid gland, producing the thyroid hormones T1, T2, T3, and T4. An *iodide* is a compound of iodine that contains another radical or element, such as potassium iodide. T1 has one iodide molecule attached, T2 has two iodide molecules, T3 has three, and T4 has four iodide molecules.

A picture may help you to visualize how the thyroid hormones actually look. Figure 3.1 shows a simplified picture of these hormones. This is how I draw them for patients during a consultation. The real biochemical structure is, however, much more complicated. The hormones are drawn this way to illustrate the point that T4 has four iodides and T3 has three iodides.

T1 and T2, as stated previously, are considered "precursors," which means they are used by the thyroid gland primarily to make the final active hormones, T3 and, mostly, T4. The gland then releases a larger amount of T4 and a small amount of T3 into the bloodstream. All four hormones are present in the thyroid gland, and as you may

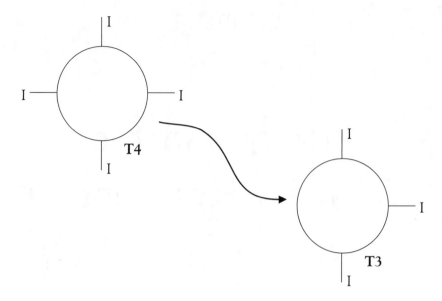

Figure 3.1: Normal conversion from T4 and T3.

remember from chapter 2, they are also present in several thyroid medications, Armour thyroid medication, for example.

These hormones are dispersed to all the other organs of the body including the skin, the liver, the kidneys, and the brain. T3 and T4 affect metabolism. T1 and T2 are not released in the bloodstream but are, instead, recycled in the thyroid gland to make more T3 and T4 in the future.

Peripheral Conversion of T4 into T3

T4 is the main thyroid hormone produced. It is sent into the bloodstream where it is converted, to a degree, into T3, which is several times more active metabolically than T4 is. This conversion from T4 into T3 is a very important step that sometimes doesn't take place as it should due to various factors, such as aging, genetics, stress, and various deficiencies of vitamins and minerals. Chemicals, heavy metals, and medications also can affect this peripheral conversion of T4 into T3.

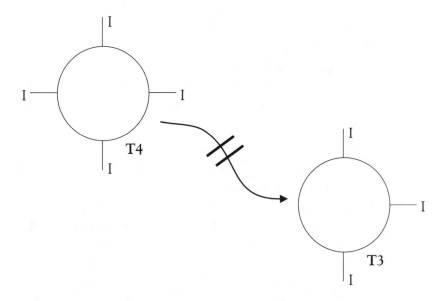

Figure 3.2: Blocked conversion from T4 and T3.

Now, take a look at figure 3.2 showing the same wheel shape, but in this illustration, the conversion is being blocked. The horizontal lines cutting across the arrow represent a blockage affecting the action of an enzyme called deiodinase. The presence of this enzyme is responsible for cutting off one of the iodide molecules (the spokes on the wheel in figures 3.1 and 3.2), creating T3.

The T3 hormone then attaches to the cells of the body and enters the cells, thus turning on the cellular energy–producing process.

THE CELLULAR ENERGY–PRODUCING PROCESS

Now, let's take a look at what we mean by cellular energy or the cellular level.

- The hormone T3 attaches to the cells at receptor sites. T3 then enters the cells and goes directly to the nuclei of those cells where it interacts with other receptor sites. Once these receptor sites have been activated by T3, signals are sent to the cellular "machinery" that uses the chemical and molecular constituents of food to produce energy.

■ The cells make energy inside these structures that are known as *mitochondria*. Mitochondria are small structures within the cells that produce the enzymes necessary for energy production.

■ The Krebs cycle is a biochemical process by which the food materials are burned up and packets of energy are released and made available for each cell to use. This process is influenced by thyroid hormones. A person with a low thyroid will make less of this energy and will therefore be more tired. The process then becomes an unending cycle that continually breaks down the body functions further and further. If you can't make much energy, then you have less energy to use, you make even less energy again, and the cycle can go on and on until the root of the problem is addressed and corrected. That is why, clinically, I consider the thyroid hormones to be the "hormones of vitality."

Various nutritional substances, such as vitamins, minerals, and fatty acids, are needed to facilitate the final step of the thyroid hormone attaching to the cells and entering into the nuclei of the cells. Note that someone who has suffered from a chronic illness for several years would have difficulty being able to utilize the thyroid hormone, even when replacement medication is administered.

In chapter 1, the subject of jump-starting the thyroid was discussed as was the need for adjusting and fine-tuning the dosage of any medication. This is because some people have spent years barely functioning because of a low thyroid that has burdened the rest of their body's reserves. Such a burden throws off the entire biochemistry of the body, lowering the resistance against disease and causing every other natural mechanism to function badly. The body that has experienced a chronic condition of low thyroid can be likened to a rusty engine in that once it's unclogged and responding to the effects of the thyroid hormone, it can function like new.

Thyroid Treatment Resistance

Consider someone who has had rheumatoid arthritis for a number of years. After appropriate clinical evaluation and testing, the patient is started on thyroid replacement therapy. There is no immediate response. That person's system is so clogged up, so backed up from years of toxins, nutritional deficiencies, or external stresses, that the thyroid hormone is prevented from taking effect right away. So, when that patient returns to his or her doctor for reevaluation a month later, no improvement will be reported. That person's thyroid is like a dead battery that cannot be jump-started even though the warranty has not expired.

Speaking clinically, I have seen this numerous times over nearly thirty years of practicing medicine. Over the first few months, some patients report back that they feel nothing, no improvement. Then, by the third month of treatment, as the appropriate dosage is finally found, that dose of thyroid replacement hormone is able to penetrate the clogged-up machinery of the body, and the treatment finally kicks in. Then the patient suddenly says, "Wow. I feel better!"

Why is that? Years of being sick with a low metabolism and with debris collecting in the cells act like a blockage in the whole system. The thyroid replacement therapy works like kick-starting an engine, clearing the debris out of the cylinders. What do you think becomes of all those years of waste products, of constipation, lack of activity, and lack of circulation?

In a healthy body, like a well-maintained engine, the waste materials are supposed to be excreted efficiently and regularly: from the skin by sweating, from the bowels by defecating, from the waste products of the kidneys that are passed in urine, and from the lungs by breathing. If they are not excreted in these ways, the waste builds up and creates a clogging of debris that interferes with the working of the thyroid hormones, at least initially. Thyroid replacement therapy does work; but for people with chronic health conditions it is quite likely that the healing processes will take some time to become activated, and even more time to work through the cells to rejuvenate the metabolism, the process by which energy is created.

Catabolic vs. Anabolic Hormones

I consider the thyroid hormones to be "cleansing hormones" because they are essential in helping the body to rid itself of the buildup of debris by restoring both the metabolism and the circulation to healthy levels of activity. So, unlike other hormones, thyroid hormones are *catabolic,* which can be understood as another word for cleansing, inasmuch as they break down debris and help to rid the body of waste matter. Many other human hormones are *anabolic,* which means they enhance tissue growth by building up matter, whereas thyroid, a catabolic hormone, breaks matter down and cleanses the body.

Myxedema

The term myxedema, coined in the late 1800s, is the name given to severe cases of hypothyroidism. *Myxedema* is characterized by thickness of the skin and general puffiness, along with other low thyroid symptoms. The thickening of the skin and other symptoms are resolved with thyroid hormone treatment. Have you ever seen "before" and "after" photographs of people with severe hypothyroidism? These "before" photos show people with extreme overweight puffiness. The puffiness shows itself in the face and as weight gain and swelling or edema in the body. The "after" photos show the symptoms resolving over the course of a year. It is quite amazing to realize that these photos are all of the same person. In the initial photographs, the people look extremely dull and sluggish; in the later photos, when the people are well into thyroid treatment therapy, they look much livelier and much more fully alive. Clinically, in the office, we see this with patients who change dramatically as their thyroid treatment progresses month by month. Some patients return to being their former selves, the person they remember being long ago. In other cases, the patients blossom into totally new, sparkly, animated version of themselves.

T3 AND THE CELLULAR PROCESS

It is the T3 that actually turns the cellular process of restoration back on. It is essential to have enough T3 to optimize its effectiveness in terms of making the cells work properly, which means they can accomplish their constant job of turning food nutrients into energy as effectively as possible. Because T4, also known as *thyroxine,* is converted into the more powerful T3, sometimes T4 is considered a "prohormone," meaning a precursor or "mother" hormone, whereas T3 is considered to be the more active hormone.

Maximizing T3

Since T3 is the thyroid hormone that gets the job done, it's crucial to be sure you are taking enough T3. It's also important to take other natural supplements that help to support the thyroid gland's activity. As stated earlier, the thyroid gland is necessary for health and vitality; this fact cannot be repeated too often because it is essential for your health and well-being to understand the role your thyroid gland plays in your overall functioning.

Thyroid Hormone Resistance

What happens when your thyroid gland malfunctions and cannot produce enough T4 or T3? Over time, you would begin to notice that your ability to function well in the world has deteriorated. You might observe that your short-term memory doesn't work as well as it used to. You can't remember people's names. You can't multitask. When you try to do too many things at once, you become overwhelmed very quickly. You might become prone to weepiness and cry very easily. You might become depressed. This can be quite serious. If your thyroid problem goes undetected and untreated, you could lose your job. You might have to go on disability leave, and you could sink even deeper under a cloud of hopelessness and depression.

What happens if your body simply cannot convert the T4 into T3? What if the T3 has trouble entering the cells and turning on your cellular metabolism? The key point about these thyroid hormones is this: If your body doesn't get T3 to your cells in a usable way, you are going to have a lot of seemingly unsolvable problems due to exhaustion, poor concentration, weight gain, and depression.

This particular combination of exhaustion, inability to concentrate, weight gain, and depression could be due to thyroid hormone resistance. There are, in my experience, degrees of partial thyroid hormone resistance in patients. So, it isn't all or none. That is, the symptoms listed above are expressed in differing degrees of severity. Especially in chronic diseases, the thyroid receptors on the cells may become damaged or blocked, preventing thyroid hormone from attaching to the cell and entering into the cell in sufficient quantity.

According to Alan Gaby (2003), these problems with the receptors can arise from genetic tendencies or from damage to the receptors caused by an autoimmune or oxidative mechanism. Also, other chemicals can bind to the thyroid hormone receptors (Brownstein 2002). So, if the body cannot convert T4 into T3 on its own as part of the natural process or if enough T3 is not able to attach to the cells due to thyroid hormone resistance, an individualized treatment protocol must be created and implemented to provide the quantities of each necessary for that patient's optimal functioning. But first, let's go on to the causes of hypothyroidism in chapter 4.

Summary

■   The thyroid gland is essential for health and vitality.

■   All four thyroid hormones, T1, T2, T3, and T4, are present in the thyroid gland.

■   T1 and T2 are precursors.

■   T4 has four iodides. T3 has three iodides.

■   T4 is the main thyroid hormone produced. It is the "mother" hormone.

■   T3 is the "action" hormone.

■   Thyroid hormones are the hormones of vitality.

CHAPTER 4

The Causes of Hypothyroidism

There are several reasons why people become hypothyroid. A low thyroid condition can occur gradually, in degrees, from very slight to worse degrees of thyroid failure. These different grades have been described as grade 4 (the presence of antithyroid antibodies without any other laboratory abnormalities present), to grade 3 (subclinical hypothyroidism), to grade 2 (mild hypothyroidism), to grade 1 (overt hypothyroidism). These different grades of hypothyroidism can result from any of several causes that are discussed below.

A TIRED THYROID

Often the thyroid gland doesn't make enough thyroid hormone on its own. This is a common occurrence; this condition is called a "tired" thyroid. In these cases, there is nothing overtly diseased about the gland. It just doesn't work well enough for some reason and, often, that reason is not found. To be practical, these patients do respond well to thyroid replacement therapy and they do feel better.

In traditional endocrinology, whether the tiredness results from the thyroid itself, from the pituitary gland or the hypothalamus, or whether it is related to other factors, typically, the bottom line is that giving the patient thyroid replacement therapy corrects the deficiency and the patient feels better. As will be discussed in chapter 7, there are other more nutritional approaches to rejuvenating a tired thyroid gland that can be added to the treatment, or even used as a main treatment in mild cases.

Hashimoto's Thyroiditis

The autoimmune disease called *Hashimoto's thyroiditis* (also called thyroiditis) is another main category of hypothyroidism. In this disease, for reasons that are not clear, the thyroid gland is attacked by the body's *lymphocytes* (a type of white blood cell) causing an inflammatory response. The inflammation can result in either hyperthyroidism or, after a certain burnout period, a low thyroid. During the burnout period the thyroid gland is attacked by lymphocytes, weakening the thyroid's ability to make thyroid hormones. In these cases, the patient's blood tests will show the presence of an abnormally high level of thyroid antibodies, specifically antiperoxidase antibodies. Moreover, a biopsy of the thyroid gland will show an infiltration of lymphocytes in the thyroid tissue.

In Hashimoto's thyroiditis, the gland is not able to function normally and may become diffusely swollen and tender. The normal process of making thyroid hormones is upset, and, in these cases, adding extra iodine to the diet can often make things worse. Normally, iodine, found in a seaweed-like kelp, for example, is recommended to stimulate the thyroid gland in cases of low thyroid. In cases of thyroiditis, however, the iodine can cause the gland to swell and become more tender. In many low-grade or chronic cases of thyroiditis, the gland is neither obviously swollen nor tender at all. In many cases, the patients don't even know they have thyroiditis.

In some rare cases of thyroiditis, the actual thyroid antibodies may not be present, although this is the way thyroiditis is usually diagnosed. Then, an ultrasound of the thyroid gland may be ordered and it will be abnormal, which is consistent with a lymphocytic infiltration. In such rare cases, a biopsy of the gland may be required for proper diagnosis.

A TYPICAL PATIENT WITH HASHIMOTO'S THYROIDITIS

Often a typical patient with thyroiditis will come into the doctor's office complaining of tiredness and seeking a thyroid evaluation. After the appropriate blood tests, the thyroiditis is then discovered for the first time. Often, this is discovered after years of the patient being told that his or her thyroid was normal. Upon review of the patient's medical records, the doctor finds that a blood test for thyroid antibodies was never done. So, the first way of determining whether a patient has Hashimoto's thyroiditis is through a thyroid antibody test, which may be followed up with a thyroid ultrasound. (See chapter 6 to learn more about step-by-step testing methods.) So, to summarize, Hashimoto's thyroiditis is one of the main causes of hypothyroidism.

According to Hendrick, Altshuler, and Whybrow (1998), even subtle abnormalities like the presence of thyroid antibodies can produce neurobehavioral symptoms, such as depression and subtle cognitive memory, concentration, and focus problems. Patients with antithyroid antibodies are at a high risk of progressing to overt hypothyroidism. Among patients with mild hypothyroidism who have these thyroid antibodies, 80 percent of them will progress to a worsening of their thyroid condition within four years (Surks and Ocampo 1996).

Other immune system–related antibodies exist that can be abnormally elevated and can affect the thyroid. These antibodies include TBII and TBA, which are less well-known than the antibodies for Hashimoto's thyroiditis and, usually, doctors do not order these tests when evaluating hypothyroidism. TBII and TBA can be elevated, and I have seen cases where the patient does have low thyroid function and, finally, these other abnormal antibodies are found. This points to an imbalance between the immune and endocrine systems relating to the hypothyroidism. The treatment, then, might take this imbalance into consideration, not only in terms of prescribing thyroid hormone but also in working to improve the immune system.

NODULES

Other cases of low thyroid can be detected at the doctor's office because the patient has a specific lump or multiple lumps or nodules on his or her thyroid gland, a *goiter* (an enlargement of the thyroid gland), or a multinodular goiter. These patients could be either hyperthyroid (overactive) or hypothyroid (underactive or low), and the size and nature of their lumps should be checked. For this reason, an ultrasound or a biopsy of the thyroid gland should be done to determine whether the nodules are benign or malignant.

If the goiter is benign, it very often responds to thyroid replacement therapy. Sometimes, however, it may not respond or the situation may not be clear, in terms of the presence of malignancy, and in these cases, the patient has surgery or undergoes a radioactive procedure to destroy the thyroid gland. This, of course, gets rid of the nodules but it also gets rid of the entire thyroid gland permanently. Those patients then must take thyroid hormone replacement therapy for the rest of their lives.

OTHER CAUSES OF THYROID DYSFUNCTION

Regarding these basic types of low thyroid conditions, eventually the question is asked as to what else might be going on to contribute to the development of hypothyroidism. In other words, as you'll see in chapter 6 on testing, we might get the thyroid laboratory results and then see that although the thyroid is low, there is no obvious disease such as thyroiditis present.

A doctor might tell the patient that her or his thyroid hormone levels are below normal, but that no thyroiditis is present and there are no lumps in the thyroid gland itself. Then, the doctor might say something like, "Let's just give you some thyroid replacement therapy to alleviate your low thyroid condition." However, it is my belief that the doctor should also look for the real root cause of the low thyroid.

Deeper Causes of Thyroid Dysfunction

The point is that, along with a thyroid replacement prescription, as you'll see in chapter 7 on treatment, you'll also want to be made aware of the other root cause or causes, in order to effect a real recovery of your health. Now, let's discuss some of those other causes.

IODINE DEFICIENCY

An iodide is a compound of iodine that contains another radical or element, such as potassium iodide. Iodide, which was defined in chapter 3 as a compound of iodine, is also called "ionic." In this book, you will see the terms used interchangeably.

Certainly, in parts of the United States, such as the areas far away from either the Atlantic or Pacific oceans, people who chronically did not get enough iodine in their diets frequently did develop large benign goiters. In fact, those parts of the U.S. were once called "the goiter belt" (Wright 2002). According to a review article, the average person needs to get approximately 60 micrograms (mcg) of iodide a day to give the thyroid gland enough building blocks to make the thyroid hormones (Kelly 2000). If you don't get enough iodide, you will experience a deficiency of thyroid hormones because your gland won't be able to make enough. In some cases, the gland enlarges over time, producing a goiter. In many cases I've seen in my practice, there is no obvious enlargement, but the levels of T3 and T4 are low. Sometimes giving iodine to the patient does help to raise these levels, but that doesn't work for everyone.

HEREDITY

It has also been my clinical experience that heredity plays a role in many cases. I've found that the tendency to low thyroid runs in families. For example, in my practice, I've had one patient and that patient's mother and several aunts all on thyroid replacement therapy for treatment of low thyroid.

Today, there are tests available that test for genetic predispositions to various conditions and illnesses. However, these genetic tendencies don't always manifest themselves clinically until other stresses or nutritional deficiencies become involved. So, someone may have a predisposition to hypothyroidism but be absolutely fine until reaching his or her forties. Then that person may go through a period of stress and become hypothyroid.

It is interesting that often patients who have been diagnosed with hypothyroidism will slowly learn about relatives and ancestors who were also diagnosed as having low thyroid. It is even more interesting to note that many relatives of someone with low thyroid are often depressed, but they have never been tested for low thyroid.

If you are depressed and you've been diagnosed with hypothy-roidism, at this point you can benefit not only yourself by treating your depression with thyroid replacement therapy, you also may help other family members. You can do this by pointing out to those relatives the link between thyroid and depression that may be hereditary. I have seen the family link between these two disorders time and time again, for example, with mother-daughter-aunt connections or with daughter-mother-brother.

The Deiodinase Family of Enzymes

Almost any chronic disease process, nutritional deficiency, or toxic chemical buildup can also influence the thyroid gland and the body's ability to metabolize the thyroid hormones and use those hor-mones at the cell receptor sites. The deiodinase enzymes are involved in the metabolism of T4 into T3. In a moment, you'll see why a quick overview of these enzymes is helpful for understanding why people may develop hypothyroidism. Any factors that affect these enzymes will affect the production of T3 as well as the level of rT3. (The term *rT3* means reverse T3; this is another form of T3, but it is inactive.)

The type I deiodinase enzyme is found in the liver, kidneys, and the skeletal muscles. It is the main enzyme involved in the peripheral metabolism of thyroid hormones in the body. (The term *peripheral metabolism* refers to the conversion of T4 into T3 in the body.) Type II deiodinase is found in the brain, the pituitary gland, and in brown fat. Type II is the main deiodinase enzyme of the brain (and central ner-vous system). It converts T4 into T3 in the brain. Type III deiodinase also exists in the brain and it converts T4 into rT3 only.

In some physiologically stressful circumstances, such as selenium deficiency; cadmium, mercury, or lead poisoning; an excess of free radi-cals; and chronic liver and/or kidney diseases, there can be a deficiency of T3 due to interference with the type of deiodinase enzyme that makes the T3. In cases of toxic metal exposure, the enzyme activity is reduced by up to 90 percent. In such an instance, what the clinician will want to do is to increase T3 to its optimal level and to decrease or lower the levels of rT3. However, many factors affect T3 detrimentally (Kelly 2000). Let's take a look at a list of some of the factors that con-tribute to a decrease in T3 and an increase in rT3.

Factors Known to Decrease T3 and Increase rT3

- Burns

- Chemical exposure

- Caloric restriction and fasting

- Alcohol excess

- Liver and kidney disease

- Diabetes requiring insulin treatments

- Stress in general

- Stress relating to critical illness

- Stress relating to injury

- Surgery

- Toxic metals

- Increase in cortisol due to stress

- Increase in inflammatory *cytokines* (messenger molecules that become elevated with inflammation)

- Some medications (propranolol, amiodarone, dexamethasone, and possibly other drugs)

- B_{12} deficiency

- Zinc deficiency

- Selenium deficiency

SELENIUM, T3, AND RT3

Selenium is definitely required for the type I deiodinase enzyme to work properly. Remember, the deiodinase enzyme does its work in the liver, kidneys, and muscles to make T3. Selenium has been well-studied, and it is now known that a selenium deficiency causes a 47 percent reduction in the activity of this vital enzyme. This enzyme, once again, is responsible for converting T4 into T3 in the body.

Selenium is the mineral that is necessary for the type I enzyme to work; the enzyme also breaks down rT3 into its degradation products (T2 and T1). If this enzyme is compromised by any of the factors listed in the bulleted list above, a deficiency of T3 will occur and a buildup of rT3 will result. T3 is biologically active; rT3 is not biologically active. *Biologically active* means that the T3 can cause the cells to produce energy. If a deficiency of T3 develops with an increase of rT3, you will feel tired and depressed. The rT3 is believed to block the further conversion of T4 into T3.

ZINC DEFICIENCY

Zinc deficiency can also cause a decrease in T3. The level of the deiodinase enzyme decreased by 67 percent in animals who were deficient in zinc. The exact mechanism by which zinc deficiency causes this enzyme inactivity is not completely understood.

VITAMIN B_{12} DEFICIENCY

A vitamin B_{12} deficiency in animals has also been shown to interfere with the conversion of T4 into T3 by affecting the deiodinase enzyme, resulting in lower T3 levels (Kralik, Eder, and Kirchgessner 1996).

BLOOD COAGULATION

Some patients have a tendency toward a thickening of their blood, a coagulation disorder, that can result in blood clots. In milder cases, however, the patients may not develop blood clots but may develop an increase in blood *viscosity* (thickness). This increased viscosity, in turn, can slow down and reduce the blood flow to the organs, including the thyroid gland. According to Brownstein (2002), such coagulation tendencies can affect thyroid function. If, on repeat testing, evidence of a coagulation disorder is found, there are treatments that can be specifically targeted to open up the circulation.

SOY

In a study of thirty-seven healthy adults who were fed 30 grams of soybeans daily, approximately one-half of the subjects developed low thyroid symptoms after three months on the diet. Their specific symptoms included malaise, sleepiness, and constipation. Then the soy was removed from their diet, and after one month of not eating soy, all of the subjects' symptoms were resolved. There is some thought that soy may interfere with the conversion of T4 into T3. Based on animal and human studies, however, there may be other mechanisms involved

(Stangl, Schwarz, and Kirchgessner 1999). Nevertheless, soy ingestion could be a problem for patients with a tendency toward a weakened peripheral enzyme system, meaning patients who may be dealing with any of the factors listed in the bulleted list above.

HIDDEN INFECTIONS

When looking for the deeper causes of thyroid and depression, assorted hidden bacteria, fungus infections, and viruses that can upset the immune system and weaken different organs should be considered and ruled out, especially when the bigger picture of the problem has not been completely resolved with the testing and treatment of the more obvious causes. We'll discuss these possible causes of thyroid dysfunction and depression in later chapters, but for the moment, it's good to be aware of these possible culprits.

STRESS INTERFERES WITH T3 PRODUCTION

So? What does this all mean to you? As stated previously, T3 is the crucial thyroid hormone for getting the body going metabolically. Your body needs sufficient amounts of T3 for energy, metabolism, and for living an energetic life. Any kind of acute stress can interfere with the deiodinase enzyme and subsequently cause a lack of T3 in the body and a buildup of rT3.

So many people who come to see me in my office complain about the stresses of modern life. As it turns out, these stressed-out patients also frequently experience many of the symptoms listed under Signs and Symptoms That May Indicate Hypothyroidism in chapter 1. Although some patients suspect that they may have a low thyroid, others are simply looking for answers and relief from what they think may be, for example, a case of heavy metal poisoning, or fatigue, or depression. So, if you use the bulleted list above, Factors Known to Decrease T3 and Increase rT3, in conjunction with the list of signs and symptoms from chapter 1, you may be able to identify some clues that will help your doctor diagnose your condition more accurately. When you look at your body from a holistic, metabolic perspective, you can see there are many causes of depression. Then, as you'll see when you continue reading, we will discuss understanding and solving the roots of depression.

Summary

Hashimoto's thyroiditis is one of the main causes of hypothyroidism. Other causes of hypothyroidism include iodine deficiency, hereditary influences, and hidden infections.

Other factors affect the actual production of the hormones in the thyroid gland, and what happens to the hormones in the peripheral metabolism. Peripheral metabolism refers to the conversion of T4 into T3 and reverse T3, and to how these T3s are subsequently broken down further into T2. Factors affecting conversion include heavy metal poisoning, stress, and deficiency of key minerals and vitamins. Symptoms should not always be seen as just symptoms but more as clues, to get to the root problems that must be addressed before the patient can experience true healing.

CHAPTER 5

How Thyroid Function Affects Depression

WHAT WE KNOW ABOUT THYROID FUNCTION AND DEPRESSION

The purpose of this chapter is to expand your knowledge about depression and its link to hypothyroidism. The medical community has known for more than fifty years that there is a link between the thyroid and mental and emotional well-being. It has been recognized for many years that a low thyroid state is often associated with depression. This was discussed by Broda Barnes in his book *Hypothyroidism: The Unsuspected Illness* (1976) and goes back much further to an article written about low thyroid by R. Ashner in the *British Medical Journal* in 1949.

During the past twenty years, the increased variety of available prescription antidepressants combined with a greater cultural awareness of depression has prompted more patients to report that they are depressed. This higher incidence of reported depression has compelled doctors and patients to rely on antidepressants as a main treatment option. The convenience and ease in prescribing antidepressants made sense in an era of HMOs, pharmaceutical companies' research, and patients' desire for the quick fix. All of these reasons escalated the widespread use and acceptance of antidepressants as the only treatment for depression. It was hoped that antidepressants could be prescribed to fix the problem rapidly, and thus allow patients to lead productive, nondepressed lives.

In addition, various prescription drug antidepressants were developed based on contemporary research on the neurotransmitters involved in depression. However, in the last several years, there has been a resurgence of interest among clinicians into the link between the thyroid and depression. Currently, according to Arem in *The Thyroid Solution* (1999b), "We are witnessing a surge in interest among psychiatrists in using and reassessing T3 as a medication to treat depression in conjunction with conventional antidepressants" (page 106).

What Is Depression?

It might seem there is a simple answer to the question "What is depression?" but today when there are so many classifications, subtypes, and degrees involved in diagnosing depression, it can be confusing for a patient to understand a diagnosis of depression and what it means in terms of his or her life. The key question is this: If you are depressed, what do you need to know to pull out of your depression so that you can continue to go on and thrive in your daily life?

In previous chapters, you've learned all about the thyroid gland and how it works. In later chapters, you will learn about the subtleties required to make a low thyroid diagnosis and the complex testing that must be done to understand the complete picture of thyroid health and what that means in terms of the many symptoms you often find yourself juggling.

Since most cases of hypothyroidism go undiagnosed, it's difficult to state an exact percentage of how many depressed patients also have a low thyroid. Subclinical hypothyroidism tends to predominate in women and occurs in approximately 7.5 percent of women and 3 percent of men, as noted by Hendrick, Altshuler, and Whybrow (1998). Older women, however, are at a higher risk. They are estimated to have subclinical hypothyroidism 16 percent of the time. In one study

(Gold, Pottash, and Extein 1982), psychiatric patients with severe depression were admitted to a psychiatric hospital and 15 percent of those patients also had low thyroid.

In my clinical experience, the percentage of patients with both depression and hypothyroidism in the general population could be tripled or even larger. It simply makes sense to embark on further understanding of hypothyroidism and depression diagnoses and then, importantly, to understand how the link between depression and thyroid is established. Finally, it will all begin to come together as you understand the real link and thus the real hope that exists in treating an underactive thyroid in order to also treat depression.

People who are depressed may sometimes complain that they feel sad or moody, but often they just feel that they have lost all interest in life in general. These depressed feelings can be short-lived or last a long time, even long after the initial cause or set of circumstances that triggered the depression is gone. Some patients report that after enduring four or five setbacks, major stresses, disappointments, shocks, or negative surprises, finally, they are unable to bounce back mentally and emotionally. Essentially, they lose the ability to stand up after repeatedly being knocked down. They then become depressed.

FINDING THE LINK BETWEEN THYROID AND DEPRESSION

Recent studies strongly support and document the link between depression and hypothyroidism. One study (Sender et al. 2004), for example, reported that in older patients with hypothyroidism, 38 percent had symptoms of depression. According to a study conducted in France (Sintzel, Mallaret, and Bougerol 2004), in patients with difficult depression resistant to standard antidepressant drug therapy, 52 percent were found to have hypothyroidism versus only 5 percent in the general population. According to an important article published in the United States (Henley and Koehnle 1997), 100 percent of patients with severe hypothyroidism also suffer from depression. This is a subject of increased interest that is gaining momentum. I am sure that more articles and studies in the medical literature will explore this link between low thyroid and depression.

Are You Depressed?

In some instances of depression, patients will eat more and gain weight. In other cases, they will lose their appetite and lose weight. In some cases, they sleep more; but some patients experience great difficulty sleeping and too-early-in-the-morning awakening. In many cases of depression, they will feel tired or will develop unpleasant bodily sensations, such as aches and pains, headaches, decreased sexual drive, and lack of interest in sex. Sometimes, depressed patients are aware that they are depressed in that they know their mood is down and they aren't functioning well in their daily life. However, more often than not, patients notice that they just don't feel good. Although they know they are tired and may have lost their enthusiasm for life, often they don't realize they are actually suffering from some type of depression. What we've seen in clinical practice is that depression is a big problem and there is definitely an association with low thyroid. Now, let's take a look at the signs and symptoms of depression.

THE SIGNS AND SYMPTOMS OF DEPRESSION

Patients' characteristics when they are depressed are as follows:

- Sad, gloomy mood
- Less outgoing, more introverted
- Feelings of hopelessness
- Fatigue and exhaustion
- Crying spells
- Irritability and increased sensitivity to criticism
- Lack of interest in life in general
- Decreased enthusiasm
- Poor memory and concentration
- Mental dullness and trouble making decisions
- Insomnia
- Hypersomnia (excessive sleeping)
- Loss of appetite
- Weight loss

- Increased appetite

- Weight gain

The Importance of Testing Thyroid Function

As you will see, if you take a look at the bulleted list Signs and Symptoms That May Indicate Hypothyroidism in chapter 1, many of the symptoms for hypothyroidism match the symptoms for depression. The point is, in some cases, it may be the low thyroid that is causing the depression. In other cases, it may be that the patient has both problems occurring at the same time. In some cases, the patient will improve with thyroid treatment only; in other cases, thyroid will be used in conjunction with an antidepressant or other natural neuro-transmitter-enhancing supplement. See chapter 7 for a discussion on treatment modalities.

There may be rare cases of depression that cannot benefit from thyroid treatment. Nevertheless, in every case of depression, it is optimal practice to test very thoroughly for thyroid dysfunction, much more thoroughly than is usually done in initial screening examinations. When the testing is thorough, then if anything is found in keeping with a low thyroid function, it is crucial to include some kind of thyroid treatment protocol in the overall treatment plan for maximum benefit to the patient.

In fact, according to Hendrick, Altshuler, and Whybrow (1998), in some circumstances, even depressed patients with normal thyroid function may benefit from thyroid supplementation. In chapter 6, we'll examine carefully the issue of accuracy in lab testing for hypothyroidism. When medical doctors say a patient has a normal thyroid, what does that mean? Unfortunately, that conclusion could be the result of inaccurate or incomplete lab testing and without a clinical evaluation by a physician who understands subtle hypothyroid signs and symptoms.

Hendrick, Altshuler, and Whybrow (1998) go on to say, "Patients with subclinical hypothyroidism are reported to have a lifetime prevalence of depression of 56 percent compared with the prevalence of 20 percent depression in euthyroid (normal thyroid) patients" (page 281). That means that if you have a low thyroid you are three times as likely to suffer from some degree of depression as compared to the rest of the population.

TYPES OF DEPRESSION

It is worthwhile at this point to list some of the most prevalent categories of depression:

- Major depression

- Low-grade depression

- Chronic depression

- Manic-depressive syndrome (bipolar disorder)

- Cyclothymic disorder

- Temporary depression

- Postpartum depression

- Dysthymia

Major Depression

Over the years, different types of depression and different subcategories of depression have been recognized clinically and given names. *Major depression* is the most serious type of depression. It can include hallucinations and psychosis and lead to suicidal thoughts. Patients with this diagnosis sometimes must be admitted to a psychiatric hospital on a temporary basis.

Atypical Depression

Based on the patient's signs and symptoms regarding appetite and sleep patterns, doctors can differentiate (as best they can) among the different types of depression. *Atypical depression* is so named because, as opposed to a typical depression characterized by loss of sleep and weight loss, in atypical depression, there is a tendency to sleep more and eat more, and often to gain weight.

Chronic Depression

Dysthymia is one type of chronic depression. It is the term used to indicate a chronic low mood that continues for two years or longer. If the dysthymia worsens, the diagnosis can be changed into another category of depression.

Cyclothymic Disorder (Cyclothymia)

Cyclothymia is a chronic depressive disorder that is akin to a milder form of manic-depressive disorder.

Low-Grade Depression

There are low-grade depressions that last for more than two weeks that are less serious than major depression. There are also even shorter temporary depressions that may last for even less time. Low-grade depression usually clears up and does not necessarily return.

Temporary Depression

Postpartum depression is a depression that some women experience after giving birth. It is one type of temporary depression. Postpartum depression can range from mild to major depression. In a study of 303 pregnant women who were judged to have normal thyroid function, 7 percent developed postpartum thyroid disorders. Of these patients, depression in 38 percent was resolved with thyroid treatment. In the six-month period following childbirth, up to 12 percent of women tested positive for thyroid antibodies. Thus, a connection has been demonstrated between the presence of thyroid antibodies and postpartum depression (Hendrick, Altshuler, and Whybrow 1998).

Bipolar Disorder

Bipolar disorder is also known as manic-depressive syndrome. The manic phase is characterized by ungovernable excitement. The depressed phase is self-explanatory. In this type of depression, the patient's mood can swing back and forth from the manic phase to the depressed phase.

Over the years, psychiatrists and researchers have used different names to describe these types of depressions. According to a Danish article (Kirkegaard and Faber 1998), these changes in nomenclature have sometimes made it difficult for researchers in the field to compare the results of articles written years ago with more recent articles describing depression and low thyroid.

None of these clinical diagnoses is written in stone, however. For example, a patient diagnosed with cyclothymia can worsen to a diagnosis of manic-depressive disorder. According to the fourth edition of *The Diagnostic and Statistical Manual of Mental Disorders*, also known as the DSM-IV (American Psychiatric Association 1994), the diagnosis of depression can shift from one type to another. A patient with minor depression can shift into major depression. Similarly, a patient with chronic depression could enter a phase of major depression. There also can be a crossover of symptoms between the categories of depression. *The main point to remember is that all the categories of depression are basically still the diagnosis of depression.* Regardless of what category it's in, it is all a form of depression. Treatment with thyroid hormone or any treatment that improves thyroid function can be helpful in all of these types of depression, from temporary mild depression through more severe and chronic depressions.

HOW BIOCHEMISTRY IS SOLVING THE CAUSE OF DEPRESSION

Today, articles are available reporting the association of low thyroid and depression detailing the neural pathways and mechanisms involved in brain function. These brain biochemistry mechanisms might explain depression from a biochemical point of view and demonstrate how these pathways are affected by thyroid. So how does a hypothyroid state influence depression? How are they connected from a biochemical, or molecular biology, point of view?

In looking at recent articles in the international medical literature, one quickly realizes that each attempt to study this connection is a complex process. Sometimes, many studies report that treatment with thyroid hormone really helps depression, but an occasional study does not show this. Then, subsequent studies refine the issue in question by using even better methods of testing and evaluating thyroid function and the degree of depression.

Why do these disparities occur as they do? It all depends on the definition of which patients are included in the category of hypothyroidism, which criteria are used to evaluate whether or not these patients have hypothyroidism, and what criteria are used in evaluating which patients are depressed and which patients are improving. Furthermore, in some studies, depressed patients are asked to fill out a self-administered questionnaire whereas in other studies more complex analysis is administered by trained staff personnel.

Depression, from a biochemical standpoint, is believed to be caused by a problem with either the adrenergic system or the serotonergic system in the brain. Some patients with depression are low in noradrenaline, the main neurotransmitter of the adrenergic system. Other research points to a deficiency of serotonin, another important neurotransmitter. This is why some depressed patients have been treated with various antidepressants, such as amitryptyline, which are in the tricyclic antidepressant family of drugs. Other patients are treated with the newer SSRI (selective serotonin reuptake inhibitors) drugs, such as Prozac.

Both of these types of antidepressants act as "uptake" blockers, which means they prevent the neurotransmitters from being taken back up again into their storage places in the nerve endings, forcing the particles of serotonin or noradrenline to remain actively involved in the synaptic space. In other words, they raise the levels of these neurotransmitters in the open spaces between the nerve endings, called the *synapses*. As these levels of the neurotransmitters go up, patients report that they feel better in terms of their mood. Patients report that they feel calmer, their depression lifts, and they are able to accomplish more. As more research is done we will probably find out that these drugs work in other ways too. There is some evidence, according to Dratman and Gordon (1996) and Mason, Walker, and Prange (1993), that the SSRIs raise the level of T3 in the brain.

Patients with depression should be tested for neurotransmitters in order to determine what their actual levels are of serotonin, noradrenaline, dopamine, and other neurotransmitters.

Unfortunately, even with the best antidepressant medications available, some patients with depression will not respond at all. According to a current article specifically about depression, only one-third of patients respond to antidepressant drugs (Costa and Silva 2005). Interestingly, according to another article in a medical journal (Joffe, Sokolov, and Singer 1995), specifically about thyroid and depression, 20 percent of patients will not respond adequately to antidepressants alone.

The administration of thyroid hormone in depressed patients has been used either alone, without any additional prescription antidepressants, or it is added to an antidepressant prescription to improve the antidepressant's ability to work. Some studies do indicate that T3 alone, without any other antidepressant, can work in some cases, but generally the thyroid hormone is added to make the antidepressant work more rapidly or it is added in resistant cases where the antidepressant has not been able to work at all by itself.

In an excellent article about thyroid and depression, twelve studies showed that T3 was effective as an augmentation or add-on therapy in approximately 50 to 60 percent of treatment-resistant cases (Henley and Koehnle 1997). A medical review (Joffe 2002) agreed, noting that in twelve independent studies, T3 augmentation was successful as much as 60 percent of the time. In a 2003 study (Agid and Lerer 2003), ninety patients with major depression were given Prozac and those that did not respond to it were given T3. The T3 was effective in ten out of the sixteen female patients who had not responded to Prozac, but, interestingly, this treatment with T3 was not effective for the men in this study.

T4 alone has also been studied to treat depression. It has been studied less often than T3 because T3 is considered to be the more metabolically active thyroid hormone. In one study reported by Hendrick, Altshuler, and Whybrow (1998), 70 percent of the women receiving T4 as augmentation therapy showed improvement compared with 20 percent of the men. High doses of T4 have also been shown to help stabilize mood in patients with rapid-cycling bipolar disorder when combined with standard medications.

THE SPECIFIC ROLE OF T3 IN DEPRESSION

The brain regulates its own supply of T3 by converting T4 into T3 in the brain using a special deiodinase enzyme found only in the brain. This fact was not known twenty years ago. The T3 levels in the brain are not directly related to blood measurements of T3 (Hendrick, Altshuler, and Whybrow 1998). In patients who have some degree of hypothyroidism, it is known that the intracellular concentrations of T3 in the cerebral cortex are reduced even if the blood levels of T3 are normal (Gold, Pottash, and Extein 1982). This is important and leads to the concept of brain hypothyroidism.

The T3 hormone is believed to act as a neurotransmitter itself and is present in large amounts in some areas of the brain that are involved with emotions. It seems to be present in large amounts around the synapses. The T4 is carried into the brain across the blood-brain barrier. Once in the central nervous system (CNS), the T4 is converted into T3. This conversion is diminished in patients who are depressed. Thus, it has been suggested that depressed patients have a central hypothyroidism that does not show up on blood tests.

Once in the brain there appears to be a feedback loop. The depression signals the hypothalamus and the pituitary glands to make more *TRH* (a hormone from the hypothalamus gland known as thyrotropin-releasing hormone) and *TSH* (thyroid-stimulating hormone, from the pituitary gland) two hormones which, in turn, signal the thyroid gland to produce more thyroid hormone. The extra thyroid hormone produced is then transported into the brain where the T3 apparently produces an increase in serotonin. In depressed patients who have a low thyroid, the thyroid may not be able to respond. Therefore, no extra T3 is produced to raise the neurotransmitter serotonin and thus to alleviate the depression. Some drugs like Prozac appear to work partly by increasing the production of T3 in the brain.

THE THREE MARKERS FOUND TO LINK DEPRESSION TO LOW THYROID

1. **Thyroid Antibodies.** There are some tests, some biochemical markers of thyroid function that have been shown to be associated with depression. The clearest marker is the presence of some kind of autoimmune response affecting the thyroid gland and the hypothalamus-pituitary-thyroid axis (HPT axis). In one Greek study (Fountoulakis et al. 2004), thirty patients with major depression were tested. All of them had high levels of TBII compared to controls. *TBII* is an autoimmune immunoglobulin that can speed up or slow down the activity of the thyroid gland. The study demonstrated that some immune system dysregulation is occurring and this affects the thyroid gland. In the same study, patients also had high thyroid peroxidase antibodies.

Again, according to the article from Denmark (Kirkegaard and Faber 1998), these same thyroid peroxidase antibodies (TPOAb) are high in patients with depression of the bipolar type and in postpartum depression. According to Sintzel, Mallaret, and Bougerol (2004), thyroid peroxidase antibodies were higher in depressed patients compared with normal patients. According to Hendrick and colleagues (1998), patients with positive thyroid antibodies have diminished thyroid gland function compared to patients who do not have antibodies to their thyroid gland. So, one of the clear markers associated with thyroid and depression is the presence of thyroid antibodies.

2. **TSH Levels.** Some studies have pointed to the somewhat high end of normal range TSH, often seen in depressed patients. In these cases, the blood levels of T3 and T4 may be in the normal range. Other articles, such as Kirkegaard and Faber's (1998), have shown that the TSH can be at the low end of the normal range in some depressed patients, but the change in the TSH level after a TRH stimulation test is not normal.

In this test, the patient's blood level of TSH is measured and then the patient is given an injection of TRH. After the injection, the TSH level is remeasured and in a normal patient with good thyroid function, the TSH level is supposed to go up. In many depressed patients, the change in TSH is greatly reduced. This is referred to as a "blunted TSH response."

In general, if a patient has a gradually failing thyroid, the TRH stimulation test will show a stronger, above-normal exaggerated response. As the thyroid continues to weaken from mild hypothyroidism to even worse hypothyroidism, the TRH stimulation test will worsen in an exaggerated manner according to Henley and Koehnle (1997). This is a test that can pick up subtle cases of thyroid failure. In patients who recover completely from depression, the TRH test returns to normal. In cases where the TRH test remains blunted, the patients are more likely to become depressed again.

3. **Elevated T4.** The third marker associated with depression is an elevated T4 level in the blood. Henley and Koehnle (1997) explained that the elevated or high normal T4 levels

seen in the blood of depressed patients may be caused by the presence of reverse T3, which inhibits the conversion of T4 into T3 in the brain. Interestingly, patients with depression who have elevated serum T4 levels are not clinically hyperthyroid but instead have low thyroid symptoms, meaning they are hypometabolic clinically.

Summary

- The link between thyroid and depression was established more than fifty years ago.

- Numerous studies have been done, and published as recently as 2005, that have further established the link between thyroid and depression.

- These studies demonstrate that depressed patients often have a low thyroid.

- Many of the signs and symptoms for depression overlap with the signs and symptoms for hypothyroidism.

- There are several types of depression and degrees of depression.

- If you are depressed, the key factor is this: What do you need to know and what do you need to do in order to go on and thrive in your daily life?

- In all cases of depression, patients should be evaluated for low thyroid.

- For depressed patients, their neurotransmitters should be tested.

- T3, although a thyroid hormone, is believed to act like a neurotransmitter. It is present in the areas of the brain involved with the emotions.

- T3 and T4 have both been studied for effectiveness in treating depression.

- There are three markers linking low thyroid to depression.

- Studies demonstrate that patients with depression and hypothyroidism experience improvement of their depression with thyroid medication therapy.

- Thyroid medication therapy should include both T3 and T4 medications.

- In all cases of low thyroid and depression, the patient should receive thyroid treatment alone or in conjunction with antidepressant therapy, if the antidepressant therapy is found to be necessary.

CHAPTER 6

Testing and
Diagnosis

THE STEP-BY-STEP PROTOCOL FOR
TESTING AND DIAGNOSIS

By now, you should have a good grasp of the connections between hypothyroidism and depression. Everything we've discussed so far is what you and I would go over in my office, if we were to meet in person. It's important for you to really understand the relationship between thyroid function and depression and how that might relate to you. Becoming informed is the first step toward healing. The best information is that which is acted upon and, in this chapter, you will start putting everything you've learned so far into action. You will also see how awareness of the subtleties in evaluating, testing, and making a diagnosis is necessary to correctly identify milder cases of hypothyroidism.

At this point, we're ready to look at testing and decide which tests may be appropriate for you to take, and we'll see which tests will be most helpful to us for determining the correct treatment for you, as we'll discuss in chapter 7. In my office I go through this process with each patient, reinventing the wheel each time by seeing each new patient as a specific individual. Because you and I can't meet in person, I've set up a step-by-step protocol for testing and diagnosis. Let's start at step 1.

Step 1

Signs and symptoms. The first step in diagnosing thyroid mal-function is to go over the signs and symptoms list in chapter 1 so that you are sure that you have these indicators. Bring this list with you to your physician so that you can go over it together. Both you and your doctor should agree that you have these signs and symptoms and that it would be prudent to conduct the correct testing to determine whether your diagnosis is hypothyroidism.

Step 2

The physical examination. Step 2 is a physical examination to check your blood pressure, pulse, knee and ankle reflexes, skin, finger-nails, hair, and the thyroid gland itself.

In someone with a low thyroid, the physical exam will show a pulse below the normal range. (The normal range is between 72 and 80.) In someone with a low thyroid, the pulse could be in the 60s.

Blood pressure can be on the low side. Normal is about 120 over 80. Your blood pressure will likely be 110 over 70 or even lower, but not always. Some people with low thyroid can even have high blood pressure. I know this can be confusing. It is just another example of how important it is to look at the subtleties of the individual's symp-toms when assessing a thyroid condition.

The deep tendon reflexes can be checked at the knees (the patellar reflex) and at the ankles (the Achilles tendon reflex). There are similar reflexes in the arms at the forearm and at the elbow. The deep tendon reflexes, especially the ankle reflex, tend to be absent or weak in those who have some degree of hypothyroidism. Instead of bouncing down and back up quickly when tapped with a reflex ham-mer, the foot, for example, moves very little or takes longer to move back to its starting position.

In someone with a low thyroid, the skin tends to be dry, especially on the upper arms and thighs or lower legs. Not only is the skin dry, requiring moisturizing lotion, but there is also a tendency to small bumps breaking out on the skin relating to hair follicles. This excess skin buildup around the hair follicles is called *hyperkeratotic folliculitis*. It is characteristic of hypothyroidism and relates to a lack of vitamin A. With hypothyroidism, the body has trouble converting beta-carotene to vitamin A and becomes vitamin A–deficient. The skin can also turn an orange color, especially noticeable at the palms of the hands and the soles of the feet. This orange discoloration, called "carotenemia," is also a due to a buildup of beta-carotene, which your body has trouble converting to vitamin A.

Upon examination, the hair will be drier, or brittle or coarse. In some cases, there is hair loss not only from the head but also from the sides of the eyebrows closest to the ears. Furthermore, the fingernails will look unhealthy. The nails will break or split or peel easily.

The thyroid gland itself is usually normal on physical examination. Sometimes, however, it will be swollen or tender. In cases of thyroiditis, it could be tender and diffusely enlarged. In some cases, there will be a noticeable lump on one lobe of the thyroid gland that is visible at the front of the neck. These swollen nodules can be felt by the doctor.

The general appearance of the patient with hypothyroidism will show at least a tendency to be overweight. Seventy percent of the patients I've seen are overweight; 30 percent are thin. Sometimes patients will have a sluggish, puffy look in their face, around the eyes. Patients with low thyroid tend to be cold, particularly their hands and feet, and they will sit in my consultation room with their sweaters and jackets on. Their temperatures run low, below 98.6 degrees.

Step 3

Keep a record of your morning temperatures. If you have more than one of the abnormalities listed in the signs and symptoms list from chapter 1, upon the physical examination I recommend that you check your temperature five days in a row to get one more valuable piece of information to help in diagnosing whether you have a low thyroid. Hypothyroid patients do tend to get cold easily, don't tolerate cold weather well, and do tend to run a consistently low temperature.

There are different methods for taking your temperature for the purpose of assessing your thyroid standing. For example, Wilson (1991) suggests taking your oral temperature during the day. The method I prefer is the one recommended by Broda Barnes (1976). It's simple: Leave a thermometer next to your bed when you go to sleep. In the morning, before getting up or moving around at all, put the thermometer under your arm for ten minutes for a mercury thermometer or less than a minute for a digital thermometer (or until the thermometer beeps).

If you are menstruating, begin taking your readings on the morning of the second day of your cycle. Men and postmenopausal women can take their temperature readings on any day of the month. Whether you take your temperature first thing in the morning or during the day, it should be taken at the same time for each of the five successive days. Normal underarm temperature is in the range of 97.8 to 98.2 degrees Fahrenheit.

If you prefer to take your temperature readings orally, follow the same procedure above, except that you will place the thermometer in your mouth instead of under your arm. Normal oral temperature is 98.6 degrees Fahrenheit. Whether you check your temperature under your arm or orally, you will obtain some useful information. In my experience, keeping a five-day record of temperature has been very helpful. It's another useful marker for piecing together a complete picture of the thyroid. Although I've found temperature readings useful, I do agree with Dr. Arem (1999c) who emphasizes the primary importance of clinical assessment and lab testing in diagnosing and treating hypothyroidism.

Step 4

First round of lab tests. These tests should include the following blood tests:

- Free T3

- Free T4

- TSH (thyroid-stimulating hormone)

- Antiperoxidase antibody

- Antithyroglobulin antibody

These blood tests are done through a local laboratory, such as Quest Diagnostic Labs, and the results are returned within a week. When you receive the results, you will have some useful information about the status of your thyroid gland. The results of the lab tests will be interpreted by your doctor along with your signs and symptoms and the results of your physical examination. All of these results must be considered together.

FREE T3 AND FREE T4

The free T3 test measures the amount of free or unbound T3 in the bloodstream. In overt or full-blown hypothyroidism, the amount of free T3 will be below normal. In milder cases of hypothyroidism, the free T3 may still be in the normal range, but it will be at the low end; that is, below the middle of the normal range.

The free T4 will also be found to be low in overt hypothyroidism cases; however, in milder cases it will still be within the normal range. It may be at the low end or even at the upper end of normal. Your thyroid gland may be making an adequate amount of T4, but if there is a blockage in converting the T4 into T3, the T4 will build up so you might actually have a situation where the T4 is at the high end of normal, not low at all.

The TSH (thyroid-stimulating hormone) from the pituitary gland will be high in overt hypothyroidism. The hypothalamus receives a signal as to how much thyroid hormone is circulating in the bloodstream. It produces TRH (thyrotropin-releasing hormone) which then goes to the pituitary gland where the TSH is made. The TSH then goes to the thyroid gland to signal it to produce more thyroid hormone.

So, in overt hypothyroidism, the circulating levels of T3 and T4 will be low due to thyroid failure. In this type of hypothyroidism, called *primary hypothyroidism,* the thyroid just can't respond to the TSH signal, so circulating levels of T3 and T4 are low, and the patient has low thyroid symptoms. (Here, *primary* means that the cause of the hypothyroidism is due to some malfunction of the thyroid gland itself.) The pituitary gland continues to produce TSH to signal the thyroid to wake up. In an overt case, high TSH means low thyroid. When this occurs, your pituitary gland is overworking to produce more TSH. The most important thing to remember about TSH results is that a high TSH actually means a low thyroid.

There are cases, however, of *secondary hypothyroidism* where the real problem is not in the thyroid gland but in the pituitary or hypothalamus. In these cases, the TSH level may be low because the pituitary gland has trouble making it. Then, because of a low TSH, the thyroid gland is not getting the signals to make thyroid hormones, so these levels of T3 and T4 will be low.

In such cases where some pituitary problem is suspected, further testing can be done to check other pituitary hormones. Also, imaging studies can be ordered, such as an MRI (magnetic resonance imaging) of the brain, to look for any small pituitary tumors.

The antithyroid antibodies (antiperoxidase and antithyroglobulin) can be normal in hypothyroidism. In patients who have a low thyroid, sometimes, there is an elevation in at least one of these antibodies, usually the antiperoxidase, and sometimes in both. This is an autoimmune problem in which the body makes antibodies against the functioning of its own thyroid gland. These antibodies can be present in both severe and less severe cases of hypothyroidism. Or they may be present alone in mild cases. In subclinical cases of hypothyroidism, the TSH is elevated but T3 and T4 are normal. In even milder cases, the patient does have subtle low thyroid symptoms but the blood tests for TSH, T3, and T4 are in the normal range. Only the antithyroid antibodies will be abnormal. However, in severe cases of hypothyroidism, the TSH, T3, and T4 will all be abnormal.

Step 5

The second round of testing and making a diagnosis. After the initial results are returned, we review the tests, remembering to take into consideration the physical signs and symptoms, the results of the physical examination, and the temperature record, so that we can put it all together to see whether a picture of low thyroid exists. Then, we might be ready to make a diagnosis and figure out a treatment plan, but let's look closely at the lab results, once again, before making the diagnosis.

If the free T3 level is truly low or at the low end of the normal range, this points to a diagnosis of low thyroid. If the TSH is above 3.0, at the higher end of the normal range, this points to a diagnosis of low thyroid. If the free T4 is below the middle of the normal range, this also points to a low thyroid diagnosis. The presence of antithyroid antibodies also indicates early thyroid gland failure. If all of these indicators point directly to a low thyroid, we can proceed with treatment right away without any need for any further immediate testing. In some cases, however, these indicators may be borderline and more testing should be done to clarify scientifically whether or not the patient has a low thyroid.

For instance, we know that in perfectly healthy young adults with no low thyroid symptoms and not on any thyroid treatment, the optimal TSH level in the bloodstream is approximately 1.5. Suppose, for example, that you have obvious low thyroid symptoms and borderline low levels of T3 but your TSH is 2.25. This would represent a subtle elevation of TSH, above the optimal level. This is an example of the kind of situation in which you would want to run further tests, such as the TRH (thyrotropin-releasing hormone) test.

The TRH stimulation test was used quite a lot years ago. Then, as other lab tests like the TSH (thyroid-stimulating hormone) test improved in accuracy, use of the TRH test decreased. For the TRH test, the patient is given an injection of TRH, and blood levels of TSH are then checked several times. In a patient with a normal thyroid, an elevation of the TSH is seen. However, in patients who are hypothyroid, the TSH response is exaggerated. In a borderline situation, this test will provide more proof that hypothyroidism exists.

Here is the second round of testing:

- 24-hour urine sample test for T3 and T4 hormones

- TBII (thyroid-binding inhibitory immunoglobulin)

For further evaluation of thyroid status, the most useful test in this list is the twenty-four-hour urine collection for T3 and T4. Obviously, this is a take-home test. After collecting your urine for twenty-four hours, you send your urine sample to the lab. The actual test is done by laboratories in Belgium or the Netherlands. This urine test uses a chromatographic process that differs from the technology used for blood tests. Its results show the levels of the T3 and T4 hormones over the course of an entire day.

When these results are returned to me, I review them with the patient. Hypothyroid patients have a truly low level of T3 and T4, both below the normal range. In cases where there is a problem converting the T4 into T3, I may see a high T4 but a very low T3. So, in this way, the urine test results are used to confirm the clinical impression of hypothyroidism. This test has been widely used in Europe for years and it is now available to patients in the United States. It takes approximately three to four weeks to receive the results of this test.

The TBII test is a blood test for immunoglobulins that can have a slowing down or blocking effect on thyroid function. This test provides evidence of some immune system–endocrine system dysregulation or abnormality. The test is not ordered routinely. If it comes back positive, it is simply more evidence that the thyroid system is not entirely normal, similar to the thyroid antibody testing. The results do not change the course of thyroid hormone replacement treatment but it's likely that other immune system supportive therapy will be recommended, which you will learn about in chapter 7.

I'd like to note here that using the twenty-four-hour urine test for T3 and T4 is the most useful method for testing those two hormones. It is much more accurate because of the chromatographic technology that is not skewed by "look alike" molecules (see below).

HOW ACCURATE ARE THYROID LAB TESTS?

In measuring the T3 level in the blood, the free T3 is more accurate than the total T3. *Total T3* is a measurement of all of the T3 in the blood. *Free T3* is a measurement of the T3 in the blood that is not bound to a protein. It is free and available to function as a thyroid hormone. However, when measuring either free T3 or total T3, there are some "look alike" molecules recorded by the blood-testing equipment that can lead to a degree of overcounting the actual amount of T3 present.

The error factor is worse with total T3 measurements and better with free T3 measurements, but it is not perfect. That's why doctors will try to always use the same laboratory or even keep lab equipment in their own office to do the testing themselves. They want to minimize the error factor (or, at least, to factor in the error ratio with which they become familiar). The same error problem occurs with measurements of free T4 and total T4.

TSH (thyroid-stimulating hormone) is measured using an antibody that binds to one of the chains that comprise TSH. Unfortunately, as a rule, there tends to be an error factor in the TSH measurements that also leads to the reporting of TSH as being lower than it really is.

The most costly antibody available for thyroid testing is a monoclonal antibody that accurately binds to TSH. However, due to its cost, it is not used as often as a more affordable polyclonal antibody. The polyclonal antibody does bind to TSH but it also binds with other hormones in the body such as FSH (follicle-stimulating hormone). This results in the final value of the thyroid-stimulating hormone (TSH) being reported as lower than it really is.

Physicians who understand that thyroid function lab tests have certain limitations rely on lab values as well as on their clinical judgment (Mazzaferri 1989). If you know that the tests may be inaccurate to some degree, what can you do about this? You take into account all of your signs and symptoms (see chapter 1) and you become more attuned to your day-to-day symptoms.

No blood test can completely and accurately reveal how much of the thyroid hormones is actually reaching the cells, entering the cells, and successfully turning on the energy-producing biochemistry of the cells. This is why it is vital to develop an awareness of the subtleties of your physical, mental, and emotional symptoms. Then, you put your whole picture together with all of the information gleaned from your tests to determine whether a clinical trial of thyroid medication is warranted.

Finally, when we have low thyroid hormone results from the first and second round of thyroid-specific lab tests, along with the patient's signs and symptoms, clinical evaluation from the physical examination, and the patient's temperature record, we are ready to make a diagnosis of hypothyroidism. The patient is ready for a thyroid treatment plan, as discussed in chapter 7.

But first, to be completely thorough, let's take a look at the third round of lab testing. This round of testing is auxiliary testing that relates to the thyroid gland and hypothyroidism. As an informed person, your goal is to get better. It was probably a long road to discovering that hypothyroidism may be at the root of your depression. At this point, you can either go onto the next chapter for treatment options and return to this section later, or you may choose to get some idea of other testing that can be performed first. Right now, you may just want to feel better, but you will find that feeling well is accomplished in a series of stages, and the better you feel, the better you will want to feel and the more you will want to know to continue your odyssey toward great health.

The Third Round of Lab Testing

The following tests are made as the third round of testing to be absolutely sure that the diagnosis of hypothyroidism is correct.

- Adrenal function

- Male and female hormones

- Ferritin testing

- Chronic viral testing

■ Hidden bacterial infections

■ Intestinal parasites

■ Molds

■ Food sensitivities

■ Minerals

■ Toxic metals

■ Neurotransmitter testing

■ Liver detoxification

■ Coagulation

■ Antioxidant testing

■ Organic acids

■ Amino acids

These are some of the tests that come up most often for hypothyroid patients. Not everyone will need to look at all of these categories. The decision of whether or not to do any of these tests will be a matter of discussion for you and your doctor, based, of course, on your signs and symptoms and clinical evaluation.

Adrenal testing. This test is commonly measured using saliva and can also be measured using blood or twenty-four-hour urine testing. The purpose of the test is to measure the levels of *cortisol* (a hormone usually referred to as hydrocortisone) and *DHEA* (an androgenic hormone). I have found a definite adrenal-thyroid connection in low thyroid patients. About 70 percent of the time they exhibit adrenal weakness. Note that when a low adrenal condition is discovered, placing the patient on adrenal support also supports the thyroid.

Male and female hormones. Testing of the male and female hormones is absolutely vital for all patients over the age of forty. The purpose of this book is, of course, to focus on the thyroid, but these other hormones all support the thyroid and they all work together. It often makes sense to look at your hormones at this third level of testing.

Ferritin testing. Ferritin is a protein complex containing about 23 percent iron. This is a simple blood test that looks at your tissue stores of iron. It has been my experience that low ferritin levels need to be corrected with iron supplements for optimal thyroid functioning.

Chronic viral testing. Chronic virus infections such as EBV (Epstein-Barr virus), CMV (cytomegalovirus, a widely distributed herpes virus), HHV-6 (human herpesvirus 6), and other viruses attack and weaken the immune system, thus weakening the whole body.

Hidden bacterial infections. These infections can include myco-plasma (a group of bacteria that can cause infections in the lungs and the genitals and elsewhere) as well as Lyme disease. They weaken the system and cause inflammation, atherosclerosis, and systemic infections.

Intestinal parasites. Such parasites can live in the intestines for years, causing a strain on the entire gastrointestinal system. I have seen some patients with hypothyroidism do much better after they improve the health of their gastrointestinal system.

Molds. Some people are sensitive to molds and yeasts, such as candida. Molds are another group of infectious organisms. They can cause an inflammatory, allergic response.

Food sensitivities. Allergies and sensitivities to foods can cause fatigue and inflammations as well as other chronic health conditions.

Minerals. Certain minerals—selenium, zinc, and iron—need to be tested. Selenium and zinc, as mentioned in chapter 4, are directly involved in the production and functioning of T3.

Toxic metals. Lead, mercury, cadmium, and other toxic metals have a bad effect on the thyroid gland and on the conversion of T4 into T3.

Neurotransmitter testing. Patients with depression and mild hypothy-roidism may improve both conditions just by correcting and balancing their neurotransmitters. Testing is done using urine or blood.

Liver detoxification. The liver is one of the main organs involved in the conversion of T4 into T3. If you have been exposed to chemicals or if your liver is weak, the liver detoxification profile test will demon-strate this.

Coagulation. Not everyone has blood clots, but many people can have an increase in the viscosity (the state of being sticky or gummy) of their blood. This condition decreases blood flow to many organs, including the thyroid. Special tests for coagulation have been developed.

Antioxidant testing. The deiodinase enzyme (see chapter 3) is affected positively by antioxidants. The antioxidants improve membrane function, which improves the enzyme activity, which is responsible for making T3.

Organic acids. In complex cases, where the patient is already taking thyroid medication but there still is something else missing metabolically, the organic acid profile can help to uncover missing elements that have not yet been found. I have seen this test help the patient to achieve a difference in energy and health that can only be compared to the difference between night and day.

Amino acids. It is useful to check a blood or urine panel for amino acids. The amino acid tyrosine is one of the main precursors of thyroid hormones. If a patient is low in amino acids, then supplementation helps to improve thyroid function and, specifically, depression.

Summary

- Step 1 in testing and diagnosis is to become familiar with those signs and symptoms that relate specifically to you, your body, and your health.

- A physical examination can uncover low thyroid abnormalities.

- The hypothyroid patient has trouble converting beta-carotene into vitamin A.

- Keeping a five-day record of your morning temperature provides another marker for piecing together the complete picture of a low thyroid condition.

■ Lab testing is an important part of assessing a thyroid condition, along with your signs and symptoms, your physical examination, and a record of your daily temperature.

■ Lab testing for other related causes of low thyroid and depression can be examined and considered, as seems appropriate to your physician.

CHAPTER 7

Correcting Hypothyroidism: Treatment Protocols

TREATMENT POSSIBILITIES

To treat hypothyroidism, there is a range of possibilities from over-the-counter health food store products to prescription thyroid hormone medications to other treatments. For mild cases of hypothyroidism that do not involve thyroiditis (an inflammation of the thyroid gland), some people do respond to nutritional products that, typically, include some glandular thyroid mixed with iodine made from herbs. These products may work within just a few weeks but, in more severe or chronic cases, they may not work, which can be disappointing for the patient. Therefore, I usually find it is best to start the patient on prescription thyroid replacement therapy. I do, however, recommend that you take an individualized approach and fine-tune your program continually.

If you picked up this book because you suffer from depression and, in the course of reading it, you've suspected that a low thyroid might be at the root of your depression (based on your signs and symptoms), you should see your health care practitioner for a thorough evaluation and proper lab testing. If these tests are returned confirming your suspicions, I believe you would be wise to begin treatment with a prescription thyroid replacement, at least in the beginning, to effect a positive change in your life.

Some people might feel so much better they may then want to remain on thyroid replacement therapy. Others, once they feel better, will want to try a more holistic continuation of treatment. So, first, let's take a look at the choices of prescription thyroid hormone replacement therapy and treatment protocols. Then, let's also look at the array of natural over-the-counter options, auxiliary supplementation, and other therapies that can be helpful in strengthening your whole body.

Optimally, you should be evaluated first according to the step-by-step plan in chapter 6 to look for thyroid swelling and tenderness. Moreover, you should have your first round of blood testing done before proceeding with any treatment for low thyroid. You want to know what you need to treat and you want to know how low your thyroid numbers are before embarking on an effective treatment protocol.

Note: If there is any chance of malignancy in the thyroid gland, more studies can be ordered or arranged using a *fine-needle biopsy*. In this process, a very thin needle is inserted into the thyroid gland to remove a small piece of thyroid tissue for microscopic analysis.

PRESCRIPTION THYROID TREATMENT

The immediate advantage to using prescription thyroid medication is that it contains actual T4 or T3, and its dosage can be controlled in a logical way whereby the patient will begin to feel better, in some cases, right away. As the medication dose is increased and the optimal replacement dose is reached, patients almost always report that they feel much better. Their fatigue and depression disappear almost immediately as the thyroid hormone reaches the cells of their body and brain.

The thyroid medication does suppress the body's own thyroid gland from working, to some degree. This is both good and bad. It is good because the thyroid medication goes directly to the areas needing help: the brain, the internal organs, the skin, the fingernails and toenails, everywhere. All this makes you feel better so that you can work, exercise, return to your life, and have the energy and motivation to take care of yourself and your everyday needs.

I, however, have known patients who will avoid taking prescription thyroid medication, no matter how badly they are suffering with their particular set of symptoms. These patients worry about what will happen to them if their thyroid function is suppressed. It's true, as stated above, that taking thyroid hormone replacement therapy for any length of time will suppress your thyroid gland's natural ability to work, to some degree. However, and this is important, my approach supports your thyroid gland so that it can heal.

After all, if you find that you do indeed have a low thyroid, and you allow it to go untreated while you continue experiencing multiple symptoms, over time every other organ of your body will be strained and become affected. It doesn't make sense to leave your thyroid untreated or inadequately treated when prescription thyroid replacement is available and effective. I understand the concern, though, and that's why we continually fine-tune the treatment protocol, always taking your whole body into consideration. Prescription medication for low thyroid can increase your overall vitality so that you not only will feel better, you can begin to thrive in your life.

Many practitioners trained in natural medicine believe that, in theory, patients should be able to build up their endocrine system holistically. Nonetheless, this may not be possible in every case, and most patients need to feel better first, then they can explore natural methods with their doctor, once their health has been reestablished.

Usually, the worse the case, the harder it may be to really clean out and recharge the system. Patients with complex diseases such as chronic fatigue syndrome or autoimmune diseases may fall in this category. For these patients, it is critical that they follow the prescription protocol. When other complex medical problems are affecting other organs, along with the low thyroid and resulting depression, even with the thyroid replacement therapy, it can take weeks and even months for the benefits of the thyroid therapy to kick in clinically.

I'm reminded of one patient who had an autoimmune disease along with hypothyroidism who called me every week to complain that she "felt nothing." Each week, "nothing." Finally, after about two and a half months, she called to report that the treatment program suddenly began working. It was as if the thyroid treatment had finally broken through after years of a slow and sluggish metabolism.

Prescription Thyroid Replacement Therapy

There is no doubt that prescription thyroid replacement therapy can increase your health and your sense of overall vitality. The therapy's effects may be felt quickly or they may take some time, but they will take effect and they will help you to feel better.

ARMOUR THYROID

In my experience, the prescription pork thyroid called "Armour thyroid" is safe for people who need some help in getting their metabolism back to normal. Armour is the main brand that is commercially available at most pharmacies. Armour is a natural mix of T3 and T4 along with precursors including iodine, T1, and T2. Clinically, Armour works well for most people. I've seen only one case in which a patient was unable to tolerate Armour. Note that Armour thyroid does contain corn as a filler.

NATURE-THROID

Nature-throid is also pork thyroid. For those who are sensitive to corn, it specifically doesn't use corn as a filler. For that reason, it is a good alternative to Armour.

T3

Synthetically produced T3 is available in these two forms: Cytomel and custom-compounded T3. Cytomel tablets are available commercially in most pharmacies. Cytomel works effectively and releases rapidly into the bloodstream. It has a short half-life and usually has to be taken two or three times a day. In sensitive patients, it can cause heart palpitations because it is so rapidly released. For this reason, patients often do better with custom-compounded T3 because its release is gentler and slower.

T3 is available through compounding pharmacies in custom-compounded capsules and tablets in any strength and as a time-release preparation. Capsules of T3 made in olive oil tend to have a stronger effect than the slow time-release tablets made with methylcellulose. You can see how the treatment of low thyroid also can be a subtle art, requiring fine-tuning of both the treatment and the thyroid's response for optimal results.

T4-ONLY PREPARATIONS

Synthetically produced Synthroid contains only T4. It is available in numerous dose sizes and can be found in most pharmacies. Levoxyl is another brand name of synthetic T4.

Through compounding pharmacies, it is possible to get a combination pill made that contains both T3 and T4 together in any strength. First, you will want to establish your correct dose. The beauty of compounding pharmacies is that they can cater to the needs of the sensitive patient and to the subtle treatment of subclinical hypothyroidism by adjusting the doses of T3 and T4 by micrograms. The large chain pharmacies carry only commercially available thyroid doses in standard set strengths.

Treatment Protocol with Armour or Nature-throid

If the thyroid is low, the patient is started on Armour, ¼-grain, by mouth every morning, preferably on an empty stomach. One ¼-grain Armour tablet is equal to 15 milligrams (mg). Typically, the patient will increase the dosage from one pill a day to two pills a day, then three, then four tablets every morning, adding one tablet every seven to ten days. While increasing the dose, the patient closely watches to see how he or she is feeling. Some people need five, six, or seven pills every morning to achieve the full effect. Nature-throid is another brand of pig thyroid.

Signs of Too Much Thyroid

It is possible to take too much thyroid medication. The following list indicates the signs that too much thyroid has been taken.

- Nervousness

- Irritability

- Rapid heart rate

- Excess sweating

- Headache

- Feeling flushed or too hot

Although, most likely, you will not feel anything from one tablet of ¼-grain Armour a day, most patients start to feel better when they up the dosage to two pills of ¼-grain Armour a day, and they almost always feel better by the time they are taking three to four tablets of the ¼-grain Armour a day. Sensitive or older patients may need to use specially compounded capsules of pork thyroid in doses as low as 5 mg, as opposed to the standard 15-mg-size pill. In that way, it is safe to put even a ninety-year-old patient on pork thyroid and increase the dose gradually.

The average replacement dose of Armour thyroid is about 2 grains a day, which is 120 mg. Dosages above 2¼ grains are unusual. After repeat laboratory testing and clinical assessment, some patients need up to 4 or 5 grains a day. This dosage is somewhat rare but it may be appropriate if tested regularly and monitored carefully. Some people need more thyroid replacement than others do because many factors affect the body's ability to absorb the thyroid, transfer it to the cells, and then turn on the metabolism.

Armour is designed to be taken as a full dose in the morning. It is best taken on an empty stomach and at the same time each day. Frequently, I see new patients who come to my clinic for the first time after they've been on a low dose of Armour, which they've been taking for years. You may remember such a case study from chapter 1, Marcia's story. These patients report that they felt better initially on the Armour thyroid replacement, but that the good effect seems to have diminished. The key point is this: After retesting their thyroid hormone levels, we discover they are on a suboptimal dose. Then, if the dose is increased and brought up to the amount that is needed, these patients begin to feel better. So, you can see why it is crucially important to monitor the progress of the treatment protocol (Arem 1999c). For optimal results, the dose or type of thyroid or even other medications may need to be changed or adjusted.

Treatment Protocol for T3 Preparations

T3 is many times more powerful than T4. It is responsible for the action at the actual cellular level. Taking Armour, which has a mixture of T3 and T4, is the first step. However, if your body still cannot convert T4 into T3, as demonstrated by your repeat lab testing and clinical reassessment, you will need to add in a T3-only preparation.

Sometimes all that is needed of T3-only preparations is a small amount. For example, Cytomel is available as a 5 microgram (mcg) tablet. The patient could add to the standard 5 mcg tablet another half tablet in the morning and another half tablet in the afternoon. The dose can carefully be increased up to one whole tablet twice a day, and then a little higher, but always very carefully. During this time, while you are fine-tuning your optimal dose, you should work closely with and be carefully monitored by your health care practitioner. Some patients report that they feel different immediately on the very first day that they add in a T3-only preparation. The results can be amazing, instantly clearing up years of depression, fatigue, and other symptoms of a low thyroid.

Note: Some patients who are overweight by fifty pounds or more may need the immediate release effect of Cytomel to get results.

If the patient is using a custom-compounded form of T3, the dose can be made as low as 1 mcg. This dose can be similarly increased, very gradually, until the proper dosage is reached. Again, monitoring and repeat testing is absolutely necessary. The average replacement dose of T3 is from 10 mcg a day to 40 mcg a day, depending on the type of T3-only preparation used.

Treatment Protocol for T4-only Preparations

T4 (thyroxine) preparations are available commercially in the lowest dose of 25 mcg. It is also available as a 50 mcg white tablet that is free of any dyes. Most people tolerate the colors fine but, occasionally, a patient will be sensitive to every color of Synthroid or Levoxyl except the white tablet.

If patients are vegetarians or they observe specific dietary laws, they will not take Armour thyroid at all because it is made from pork. If they refuse to take Armour at all, I will start them on one 25 mcg tablet of a T4-only preparation every morning. Every seven to ten days, the dose will be increased to two tablets every morning, and then to three tablets every morning, increasing slowly and gradually, very carefully, before their blood tests are rechecked. The typical replacement dose of a T4-only preparation is 100 to 125 mcg a day.

If a patient is started on a T4-only preparation by itself, after retesting, it is very often beneficial and necessary to add in a T3-only preparation to the patient's program. The T3 is added in gradually, following the protocol described above under Treatment Protocol for T3 Preparations. But, at the same time, the patient will cut down on his or her T4 by approximately 20 percent in order to make room for the effect of the T3. In most cases, this combination of T4 and T3 works more effectively than T4 alone.

FINE-TUNING YOUR TREATMENT PROTOCOL

We've set out the basic guidelines for the thyroid treatment protocol above, but you are a specific individual and you may need to further customize your own protocol. As we've said, some people improve quickly and the fine-tuning becomes simply a matter of finding the correct dosages. You may, however, need to try Naturethroid instead of Armour, for example, or change the T3 compounded from one pharmacy for the T3 compounded from another pharmacy.

This may be hard to believe but, sometimes, the filler can make all the difference, even if you are not sensitive to the fillers. This is due to the time-release mechanism in the fillers. Sometimes, patience is necessary while you and your doctor work toward your goal of freedom from depression and other symptoms of hypothyroidism. And, although rare, an occasional patient will do best on T3 alone.

A NOTE ABOUT ANTIDEPRESSANTS

Depressed patients are often already on an antidepressant when they seek an evaluation of their thyroid. If you are currently on antidepressant therapy, there is no need to stop that therapy while you are evaluating your thyroid function or even when you embark on thyroid replacement treatment. To be sure, you should always inform your treating physician as to which medications you are taking.

I prefer to treat patients as naturally as possible and I prefer to help each patient get to the root of his or her problem. If lab testing, evaluation, clinical history, and family history indicate that anti-depressant therapy is appropriate along with thyroid therapy, that's fine, but always with the goal of strengthening the body, mind, and emotions so that medications eventually can be minimized or even discontinued. This will be a matter of fine-tuning your treatment with your physician.

Other Treatment Modalities

Other treatment modalities exist that can definitely enhance any thyroid treatment program. Since I believe in treating the whole body, once the low thyroid condition is under treatment, the next step is for the patient and physician to look at what other areas of the body need to be improved.

NEUROTRANSMITTERS

The real link between depression and thyroid function is that the T3 level in the brain acts like a neurotransmitter itself and interacts closely with *serotonin* and *noradrenaline,* the two other main neurotransmitters known to be involved with depression. Levels of both serotonin and noradrenaline have been found to be quite low in depressed people. Antidepressants raise the levels of these neurotransmitters. There are also naturally occurring amino acids that can raise and balance the levels of these neurotransmitters in depressed patients. *Tyrosine* and *tryptophan* are the main supplemental amino acids used clinically. Tyrosine helps to produce noradrenaline. Tryptophan helps to produce serotonin.

ADRENALS

If adrenal weakness is found on laboratory testing, this must be addressed. Years of stress have probably brought you to this point of fatigue, depression, and low thyroid. When stress affects the adrenal glands, you lose your "can do" ability and everything requires extra effort. If your adrenals are low according to lab testing, adrenal support will help by giving you just enough energy support to allow your body to heal. Over-the-counter adrenal supplements are available as glandular medications and as herbal extracts. Prescription *DHEA* (a steroid hormone produced by the adrenal gland), *cortisol* (a hormone of the adrenal cortex), and *pregnenolone* (a hormone made naturally in the body from cholesterol that acts as a precursor to the other steroid hormones such as DHEA and cortisol) can also be used.

Other Treatment Modalities for Hashimoto's Thyroiditis

Patients with Hashimoto's thyroiditis should examine and treat any food or environmental sensitivities they may have, and their vitamin, mineral, and antioxidant status should be optimized. *PABA*, one of the B vitamins, is specifically recommended for Hashimoto's thyroiditis and other autoimmune problems. Also it's important to address and correct any hidden bacteria, viruses, mold, yeast issues, or parasites.

Further Modalities

Once you have balanced your thyroid and you are feeling the wonderful benefits of that, you and your doctor will want to look at other areas of your health that may need further correcting relating to depression and your thyroid for you to continue to feel your best. Here are some other treatment modalities to consider:

- Gradually removing any toxic metals from the body that might be present has been shown to improve thyroid function (Kelly 2000).

- Treatment to improve blood flow to the thyroid gland and other organs.

- Iron supplementation, if the need is supported by testing, to improve oxygenation.

- Liver cleansing and support for liver function, with liver-cleansing supplements such as *silymarin* (milk thistle).

- Balancing the male and female hormones with bioidentical hormones via compounding pharmacies, as indicated by testing.

NATURAL THYROID TREATMENT OPTIONS

As stated above, there is an array of natural over-the-counter options, auxiliary supplementation, and other therapies that can be helpful for strengthening your whole body.

Nutritional Supplements

The nutritional products contain a variety of other glands, including hypothalamus, pituitary, and adrenal. I've seen these products help patients; however, it's hard to know when the patient needs hypothalamus and pituitary extracts, which have a stimulating effect on these glands, and which effect, in turn, has a stimulating or energizing effect on the thyroid. Just as the thyroid gland can become tired or underfunctioning without any disease being present, so, too, these other glands can become less responsive.

The main concern I have about suggesting treating hypothyroidism with these nutritional products is that, in a case of thyroiditis, the iodine and the glandular medications may aggravate the thyroid gland by causing it to swell and become more inflamed. In the long run, this could possibly lead to even more prescription therapy. The natural products are also a concern in the case of a goiter or benign growth (these appear as nodules or as *adenomas*, a type of benign growth) of the thyroid gland.

Nutritionists do use various forms of muscle testing, and some use electronic acupoint testing devices, to determine the need for these glandular medications. These methods are used infrequently by most U.S. physicians. Use of the electronic diagnostic methods is more prevalent in Europe. A few years ago, when I attended "Medicine Week" in Baden-Baden, Germany, I was impressed with the variety of diagnostic equipment that was in wide use.

In the same way that there are nutritional supplements to treat hypothyroidism, there are also a variety of homeopathic supplements available, containing animal thyroid that has been diluted down to homeopathic strengths. Similar homeopathic products exist in combinations. In mild cases of hypothyroidism, these products can do some good after a few weeks, but they can take longer to take effect. Some patients respond to homeopathic preparations and some do not.

Nutritional supplements come in a variety of forms:

- Sea vegetables in supplement form and in diet as seaweeds (dulse, kelp, wakame)

- Thyroid support supplements and herbal tinctures

- Homeopathic thyroid preparations

- Glandulars (medication made from glands)

Diet

The truth is that if you treat a low thyroid condition with thyroid hormone replacement, your condition will improve whether you change your diet or not. Nonetheless, it makes great sense to improve your diet to the best of your ability for optimal improvement of your overall health. A diet of fast food and excess refined carbohydrates just continues putting a strain on your body's organs to process needless debris.

Your first step would be to cut down on fake food, junk food, and trans-fatty acids (Brownstein 2002). You should also stop overindulging in sugars and artificial sweeteners. At the same time, add more organic vegetables, fruit, complex carbohydrates, and healthy protein to your diet. Be sure to drink enough water. You will be surprised at how your improved diet will enhance your health.

Physical Therapies

A natural approach to treating a low thyroid can include physical therapies. The following physical therapies can be quite helpful.

Acupuncture. Acupuncturists are especially skilled at *pulse diagnosis,* which is a method of feeling the pulses at the wrists to determine if the energy of the organs is blocked or out of balance in the body. By unblocking what are known as "meridians" that run throughout the body, the patient begins to feel better, and becomes more energetic and stronger. Usually, a series of treatments is required for longer-lasting improvement.

Yoga. Stretching in various yoga postures will not only help your body to become more flexible, limber, and strong, it will also move energy throughout your body. Specific yoga postures such as the high-shoulder stand, the "fish," the "arch," and the "cobra" are useful for improving thyroid function.

Massage. This therapy includes foot massage, and it affects acupuncture points that can affect the health of the deeper, internal organs of the body.

Walking. Walking in an athletic, hands-free style is excellent exercise for improving your circulation and, along with therapeutic yoga, walking provides an easy way for patients to begin a fitness regimen while they are implementing a thyroid replacement treatment.

Exercise in general. There is no one form of exercise for everyone. The idea is to start to move more as you feel ready, and to begin a movement program that is both therapeutic and invigorating. Right now, you want to breathe more and get your circulation moving, thus helping your body, mind, and emotions to maximize the benefits of your thyroid treatment plan.

Note: In many cases, however, low thyroid patients cannot call up enough energy to be able to exercise without some help from a prescription thyroid medication.

REPEAT TESTING AND VISITS TO YOUR PHYSICIAN

Every case is different. Some patients will have to continue monthly visits to their doctor while others may need to visit their health care practitioner less frequently, perhaps every two to three months. These repeat visits, especially at the beginning of therapy, must continue until the correct dosage of thyroid replacement is found. Once the correct dosage has been found and you are feeling better, you may need to visit your physician only once or twice a year for monitoring and subtle fine-tuning of your program.

Repeat testing is also done on an individual basis, but the rule of thumb is "when in doubt, retest." In other words, if you are not improving, or your progress is stunted in any manner, you and your doctor will redo some tests, also based on what your previous lab results have shown.

If your treatment progress is steady and your symptoms are improving, you may retest your basic first round of testing. Perhaps you should also retest the twenty-four-hour urine test after six months, and then yearly after that.

"Inspired." "Creative." "Energetic." "Outgoing." "Hopeful." "Clear-minded." These are some of the qualities my patients tell me they've regained with thyroid treatment. With information comes hope, and with hope comes the motivation for action. Recognizing the link between depression and your thyroid is the beginning of establishing a new level of health and well-being in your life. My wish for you is that now you can proceed forward toward enthusiasm, energy, and great health.

Summary

- Do lab testing before embarking on your treatment protocol so you know what you need to treat.

- There is a range of thyroid treatment modalities, from nutritional products to prescription thyroid replacement hormones.

- Usually T4 and T3 are given in combination.

- The best method for thyroid replacement therapy is to start at a low dose and to increase the dosage gradually.

- Other treatment modalities include balancing the neurotransmitters of the brain and adding adrenal support.

- It is crucially important to monitor the progress of the treatment protocol because the dose or type of thyroid or additional medications may need to be changed or adjusted.

CHAPTER 8

Body and Mind

By the time you reach this chapter, you will already have made tremendous strides in tackling your thyroid problem. You've learned what to watch out for in terms of signs and symptoms, you've gotten a better grasp of the different chemicals involved in the manufacture of the thyroid hormones by the thyroid gland, and you've learned how those hormones affect you. You've also learned about depression, including the kinds of symptoms to watch out for and the different kinds of depression that can be experienced. And, if you've had thyroid medication prescribed, you will have noticed some changes in how you are physically and how you feel emotionally. All this is great, but it may not be quite enough to get you all the way to "better" or "back to normal." Why not? Why can correcting the chemical balance not be enough?

This is a very reasonable question. After all, if an imbalance of your thyroid hormones has caused all of your troubles, correcting that balance should restore you to 100 percent of what you want to be. This is certainly a very reasonable expectation. But sadly, this is unlikely. That's because of the very close, intimate connection between the mind and the body; one that we often don't appreciate as fully as we should. And with good reason.

In medicine, for much of the last century the connection between the body and mind wasn't recognized. In fact, the two entities were considered separately. Doctors focused on whether you had a problem that was "organic" (caused in the body) or "psychic" (caused by a psychic conflict). This very simple and, in some sense, seductive dichotomy ("real" versus "in your head") has not served us very well, especially when we must consider physical issues that also have an impact on that most important of organs, the brain. And the thyroid gland (most glands, actually) has very critical feedback loops with the brain.

The brain "talks" to the thyroid gland, and the thyroid gland "talks" to the brain by releasing hormones. What's really happening is a cycle in which the thyroid gland affects the brain and "mind" (or psychological functioning). So, the whole notion of "mind" really comes down to brain functioning. Another way to think about it is that nothing happens in the mind that isn't at the same time a biological process in the brain. Even reading the sentences in this book could be said to be a simple function of the organ called your "brain," together with your eyes. It seems a little more magical than that, but that's what it comes down to. Everything that happens to you affects your biology, and your biology has tremendous impacts on how you think, feel, and act.

MIND THE GAP: BRIDGING THE BODY AND MIND

So, in order for people to really get better all the way, we have to expand our understanding of thyroid problems. The way to do this is to think about thyroid problems in a way that does justice to their complexities. Scientists use the term "biopsychosocial" to describe these kinds of illnesses. That multisyllabled word tells us that to tackle these kinds of illnesses we must consider the following three distinct domains:

1. **Biological underpinnings and physical symptoms.** These were the focus of chapters 1 through 7. This domain includes both the biological causes (not enough of specific hormones) and the consequences physically (e.g., fatigue, hair loss, sleeplessness).

2. **Psychological.** Here we need to look at our feelings (or emotions), our thoughts, and behavior. A biological issue that has

an impact on your brain will change your state of mind, and your state of mind will influence your biology, too.

3. **Social.** The combination of symptoms in the psychological and biological domains can have a negative impact on relationships and cause stress. Similarly, stress can put a significant burden on the mind and body, making physical illness more likely (see chapters 9 and 11). Many of the most difficult-to-treat medical illnesses fall into the category of "biopsychosocial," including heart attacks and cancer. People suffering from these illnesses, which clearly have a huge biological component, also experience many profound life changes, including the onset of depression and/or anxiety.

Good treatment centers for these illnesses almost always have mental health experts as part of the team that works with patients, in part, because it is well-understood that stress and emotional problems actually can cause physical problems to worsen. In heart disease, particularly, there are well-known psychological risks that increase the odds of having a heart attack. Considering the psychological aspects of medical illnesses is known as *behavioral medicine*. This approach considers not just the disease itself, but also the whole person, including his or her mental and emotional state. This holistic approach represents the current state of the art in medicine.

DEPRESSION AS A BIOPSYCHOSOCIAL ILLNESS

Depression represents a classic example of a biopsychosocial illness, in large part because it can be triggered in so many different ways. Abnormal thyroid function is one way for depression to begin, but some depressions occur in response to stressful life events (see chapter 11), or to relationship problems (see chapter 12). There are also circumstances in which the "normal" reaction might be to become depressed. For example, people living in refugee camps, who've been displaced because of war or a natural calamity, typically describe symptoms that indicate they are clinically depressed. Certainly, their symptoms are real and troubling, but in these circumstances, we would know that their problems are caused by external events, not by a brain or body-related factor.

Many of the symptoms of depression related to thyroid problems will be familiar to you by now, but let's take a look at them again:

■ Feeling sadness and loss of interest in normal activities

■ Changing appetite (e.g., eating too much or too little)

■ Changing sleep patterns (e.g., insomnia or sleeping too much)

■ Changing the rate of physical activity (e.g., moving very slowly or becoming physically agitated and fidgety)

■ Feeling tired all or most of the time

■ Feeling worthless or excessively guilty

■ Feeling unable to concentrate or make decisions

■ Having recurring thoughts of death or suicide

■ Worrying about minor matters

■ Feeling helpless and hopeless about the future

■ Feeling a decreased interest in sex

■ Feeling irritable and short-tempered

■ Crying frequently

■ Feeling socially withdrawn

■ Feeling "numb" or "empty"

■ Feeling easily overwhelmed

■ Focusing on oneself to the exclusion of everything else

■ Experiencing other associated problems (e.g., anxiety, alcohol or drug abuse)

Looking at these signs and symptoms again, and keeping in mind the biopsychosocial model, you can see that the symptoms of depression are well represented in all domains. Depressed people will notice some biological signs, that is, they experience problems with sleep, appetite, and fatigue. There are also changes in psychological functioning, especially in terms of habitual thoughts (thinking about dying or suicide, perceiving oneself as guilty or worthless), and emotional functioning (feeling overwhelmed, sad, numb). Furthermore, there are social changes (withdrawal, decreased interest in sex) that have a profound impact on depressed people's relationships (see chapter 12).

So, there's no doubt that depression shows itself in a number of ways; and given the breadth of the problems it creates, it is not surprising that treatment may require more than one kind of intervention. A recent finding shed more light on the biopsychosocial nature of depression and the interplay between the brain, the body, and the mind. Helen Mayberg and her colleagues (Goldapple et al. 2004) studied the brains of people who were being treated for depression. Some subjects received cognitive behavioral therapy (CBT), a talking treatment for depression (described in chapter 10); others were treated with the antidepressant Paxil.

Brain activity patterns in both groups differed from normal brain activity, indicating that both sets of people in the study had "depressed" brain functioning. When the brains of the subjects in both sets were scanned after their treatments, the researchers found that the antidepressant medication had changed brain functioning, something that was not surprising and, probably, even hoped for. However, CBT—the talking treatment—also changed brain functioning, which was visible in PET (positron emission tomography) scans before and after treatment. This, too, while a new finding, isn't all that surprising either.

We've known for years that CBT treats the symptoms of depression quite effectively and, of course, if people respond to that treatment, we also knew that, at some level, their brains are responding. It was not a real surprise, then, that these changes can be detected on a brain scan. What was surprising is the fact that the kinds of changes caused by the antidepressant and the CBT are quite different from each other.

CBT, in particular, seemed to ratchet up the level of activity in the front part of the brain, and turned down the level of activity in the parts of the brain that govern emotions (Goldapple et al. 2004). This tells us that both medications and talking treatments do something positive for the brains of depressed people, but they achieve these results in different ways. We are only beginning to understand what that might mean. Even ten years ago, the idea that psychotherapy can change brain functioning in scientifically observable ways would have made the person who made such a claim the laughing stock of the scientific establishment. But these kinds of findings are becoming more commonplace and are helping to break down the traditional wall between treatments for body and mind, that is, between biological and psychological approaches.

THYROID-DEPRESSION: FIGHTING ON MULTIPLE FRONTS

One of the themes to be developed in the following chapters is the need to change your view of the difficulties you have with your thyroid and moods. When a very clear biological problem triggers an episode of depression, there is the understandable desire for the problem to disappear just with medical treatment. And it isn't really fair that it doesn't. Let's say you have a variety of symptoms related to some other part of your body, your knee perhaps; and after a while, your doctor finds out that your problem is related to your kneecap. Let's also say that there is a surgical cure: your kneecap can be replaced with an artificial version. At some point after the surgery, you'd feel fine again; your knee would be as good as new and you'd return to full functioning. Why isn't it the same with thyroid problems?

The answer to that question probably has something to do with the extent to which your thyroid plays a role in your brain functioning, and because, unlike a kneecap, the thyroid gland is really a part of your entire central nervous system (CNS). You can think of your thyroid gland as an extension of your brain; change your thyroid and you'll change the way you think, act, and feel. In other words, unlike a kneecap problem, a thyroid problem is going to affect you profoundly.

Another fact to consider is that a kneecap problem might give you some pain, it might prevent you from bicycling or going bowling, but otherwise it would allow you to live your life. In comparison, depression takes no prisoners. It's a pretty ruthless disease, and one of the first things it does is to try to talk you out of the fact that something is wrong. As you'll learn, depression creeps into your mind and affects the way you perceive yourself and others, and worms its way into your relationships with others, too.

So, getting your thyroid balance right may be only the start of getting better. Certainly, it's a critical part of treatment, but it may not be sufficient to get you all the way to "all better." In fact, you may notice that once you've started on medication, the first things to change are the biological symptoms, like sleep, appetite, and physical energy. Other types of symptoms may not change as quickly; you may end up feeling impatient about what hasn't changed as you hoped it would. But think back to the kneecap example. Would you be 100 percent back to normal the day after knee surgery? The chances are good that you would not, that you would be required to follow a specific physical therapy rehabilitation plan, and that, before you could judge the success or failure of the surgery, you'd have to wait many weeks or even several months.

Why? Because, of course, you'd have to heal from surgery, but also because the body defends itself when it is injured; the parts of the body are interconnected and try to work together. Not having a properly functioning knee can stress adjoining areas of the leg, causing strain injuries. If you aren't able to use your leg, muscle atrophy and deconditioning would certainly occur. So, you'd need to gradually rebuild your strength, usually by doing graduated exercises. The success of your surgery would hinge just as much on your participation in your rehabilitation as it would on the skill of your surgeon.

This is the parallel with depression: rehabilitation and recovery are as important, perhaps even more so, with thyroid problems as they are with knee surgery. All of the effects that depression has had on your body and mind are likely to be less obvious than if you had had a simpler physical ailment. But the issues are just as real. So, the point of the remaining chapters in this book is to figure out what is going on with the other domains in your life, then to define what needs to be done and what role you can play in getting back to the life you want.

But what else can you do?

We've used the example of a physical injury to illustrate the point that getting better is, in part, about repairing the "cause" of a problem, followed by rehabilitation to rebuild strength and capacity in whatever body system was injured. Of course, with a purely physical ailment, this seems straightforward. After knee surgery, a specialist would design a series of movements and exercises for you to help this part of your body become stronger and stronger. How is this done for thyroid problems and the depression that results? In other words, what role can you play in your rehabilitation?

This is a critical question because, just as you wouldn't try to rehabilitate your knee without some expert advice and guidance, so, too, it's important to know what to do about depression. This is exactly what the rest of this book deals with in detail. We've selected areas to discuss that are critical to depression and to healing from depression. These areas are the "psychosocial" part of depression. Remember, this is in no way meant to offer solutions to all of the problems that depression can bring about. If you feel that you need more advice, or you struggle in areas that are different than those described, seek the help of a mental health professional who is an expert in recovery from depression.

WHAT'S NEXT

In the following chapters, we've carefully looked at the scientific and clinical literature on depression, and from that we've distilled four areas that, when addressed properly, seem to provide the most benefit. These are:

- Lifestyle factors

- Patterns of thinking

- Stress and problem solving

- Interpersonal relationships

In each of these areas, we will describe data from studies and practical advice derived from some of the most effective kinds of treatments for depression. For each chapter, we suggest you bring an open mind to the material, and try as best you can to be really honest with yourself. For some people, looking at themselves can be difficult. Many people suffering from depression would probably prefer just to take medication rather than change themselves or their lives. And, indeed, some people do very well on medication alone. On the other hand, some people really need to look into other areas to make real progress. As with many things in life, the more directions from which you look at a problem, and the more solutions you try, the better the final result will be.

Are you ready to change? For the kinds of strategies described in the following chapters, your attitude is half the battle; the other half is following through. Over twenty years ago, psychotherapy researchers began recognizing the importance of openness and "readiness for change" in effective treatment (Prochaska and DiClemente 1982).

Since then, dozens of studies have been done that demonstrate that even the best kind of treatment will be unlikely to work if the person doesn't recognize that he or she has a problem that needs to be addressed. Conversely, people who are actively ready to change appear to reap enormous benefits from treatment and actually experience much more symptom improvement.

Of course not every suggestion is tailor-made for every individual. What you read in the subsequent chapters may apply to you in some ways, but not in others. This is perfectly normal, and may reflect the circumstances of your own life, history, personality, and past experiences. We urge you to take all that you can from this book, and run with it. Be open with yourself about what kinds of changes might be helpful, and then give those ideas a try. There is nothing to lose, and your life to gain.

Summary

When you've been diagnosed with a thyroid condition, undoubtedly, thyroid medication and perhaps antidepressants will be part of your healing process. Nonetheless, when we consider the psychosocial parts of depression, we do arm you with different tools. Consider what you are about to read as potential tools for your toolkit, a more comprehensive way to rehabilitate yourself from your thyroid problems.

CHAPTER 9

A Balanced Life

This chapter will try to bridge a part of the long-standing gap between the functioning of the mind and body. As you've seen, this arbitrary distinction can really prevent us from fully considering how we play important roles in our own physical health and wellness. Sure, we can take whatever medication is prescribed, but we can do so much more than that for ourselves; simple things can heal and maximize the odds of staying well in the long run, both physically and psychologically.

Healthy lifestyle choices can be very simple. The issues examined in this chapter are not rocket science, and require no elaborate rituals or strict adherence to hard and fast rules. However, all of the following lifestyle choices have proven themselves to be important factors in physical and mental wellness regimens, and all of them are achievable by all of us with enough patience and perseverance. The old phrase "an ounce of prevention is worth a pound of cure" is apt here. But then what is really meant by an "ounce of prevention," especially in terms of lifestyle and physical wellness?

Anybody would trade an ounce of prevention for a pound of medication if that choice is possible. In this chapter, the discussion considers very basic lifestyle factors, everyday choices you can make that will give you the best chance of becoming and staying well. These are the choices that define that ounce of prevention. The following areas offer you ample opportunities to choose to prevent depression or to invite it into your life:

- Work and play

- Sleep

- Exercise

- Meaning and spirituality

These areas may seem obvious, perhaps even somewhat superficial. And yet each is vital for the health of our minds and bodies. All of these areas offer multiple choices for lifestyle modifications, but my aim here is not to tell you that you must do this or that. Instead, I will describe each area and then ask you to make your own choices about how you'd like to address that specific issue.

GETTING AND STAYING ACTIVE: PLEASURE AND MASTERY

The connection between our daily routines of work and play and depression has been long understood (Fester 1973; Lewinsohn 1974). This relatively simple but very important view of depression says that the expression of this illness involves a lack of reinforcement, or a lack of rewards from one's daily environment. Clearly, people who are depressed (for whatever reason, biological or otherwise) describe being in a state called *anhedonia,* which means a lack of interest in the activities that used to interest them and give them pleasure. This is a sign of depression but it also results in a change in behavior that can be quite profound and damaging. When people lose their interest or pleasure in a given activity, they tend to give up engaging in that activity. After all, why would anyone want to do anything that didn't give that person some enjoyment or satisfaction? In fact, people who become depressed seem to undergo quite a rational set of responses to such a change in their mood and to the change in how they experience formerly rewarding activities. They tend to give up the activities they used to engage in, one by one, because those activities no longer interest them or provide them with a sense of fun.

This seems to be an all but inevitable component of depression; in a way it is a rational response to depression. The bottom line is that depressed people often spend a lot of their time in ways that are neither productive nor pleasant. This has been described as a behavior limbo; that is, the passing of time with no particular activity taking place and no particular emotion being experienced, and yet the time goes by, unused (Bieling and Antony 2003). Depressed people can very quickly become stuck in that state because once they stop participating in a satisfying daily routine, there are very few other ways in which they can experience any sense of satisfaction or reward.

Behavioral Activation: A Rationale

For that reason, *behavioral activation* is a recommended treatment for people who are depressed. We know that this treatment works, and works quite well to change the symptoms of depression (Jacobson et al. 1996; Gortner et al. 1998).

Essentially, behavioral activation involves the slow, steady introduction of rewarding everyday activities that are chosen by the depressed person. This sounds quite straightforward, but, in practice, it can be fairly challenging. After all, the anticipation of enjoyment is often a strong motivator. It is what gets most of us interested in doing things. But that motivation appears to vanish during a depression. That is, people who are not depressed think about something they would like to do, and then they look forward to doing it, whether this be exercise, or having fun, or going to work.

People who are depressed look forward to few activities or events. They don't experience the kind of automatic urge to do things that people who aren't depressed do. It's important to point out that this doesn't mean that depressed people don't benefit from doing certain activities. They absolutely do benefit; they just might not look forward to doing them, and, to some extent, their enjoyment will likely be less satisfying than it was when they felt well.

So, the major question here is this: How can a depressed person recover his or her lost energy, enthusiasm, and joy of living? It can be done. But to do it means the depressed person must learn how to put "doing" before "feeling."

Just do it. If you are a depressed person, there will be times when you may not "feel" like doing anything at all, and yet once you do try a pleasant activity, you are likely to feel more energized, less discouraged, and more hopeful about what is possible. Here's a useful tip: When trying to assess whether a specific behavior or activity is worth doing, remember to take the long run into consideration. Don't do your assessment while you are engaged in actually doing the behavior or activity, just do it.

Balance. The other important aspect of the rationale for behavioral activation is balance. When left to their own devices, humans have an innate capacity to work and to play. We thrive in environments where we do things that challenge us (at least a bit) physically and mentally, followed by some timeoff in which we pursue distractions or pleasant sensations (yes, this includes both eating and engaging in sex). So, the idea behind behavioral activation isn't to saddle you with a schedule in which every moment is occupied engaging in activities because you should do them or you have to do them. Balance means that in addition to work you would have meaningful timeoff for yourself; time which you would use in ways you would truly enjoy.

WORK AND PLAY

There are two types of rewards we get from doing things: a sense of pleasure and a sense of mastery. Put simply, pleasure is "play" and mastery is "work." But this may be a bit too simple to help us answer the question, How can a depressed person recover his or her lost energy, enthusiasm, and joy of living?

Sometimes, the things we must do to get paid for our work, our jobs, don't provide us with a sense of accomplishment or mastery. That's because the sense of mastery results from the feeling that we can control things, and that we are accomplishing something, even if it is something quite modest. For example, the simplest sense of mastery might result from doing the dishes or the laundry. Neither task is a very grand event, but there is no doubt that when you wash the dishes, you've succeeded at changing dirty dishes into clean ones. There may not be any pleasure in doing this at all, but that is the point; it isn't fun but it does achieve something.

In fact, some mastery activities may not be much fun at any given moment. It can be challenging to plant and maintain a garden, or to change the oil in your car, but once done, these tasks become achievements. Our paid work doesn't always allow us to achieve a sense of mastery because often we can't control the activities in our work environment. So, it may be hard to measure progress in the context of your job. In many jobs there is always more work to be done and it's hard to feel that you've ever really finished something. So, just because someone is working does not mean that the person experiences a sufficient sense of mastery in his or her life. However, there are other kinds of mastery that are more personal and perhaps more rewarding. Hobbies, sports, and volunteering for the good of the community often become sources of mastery for depressed people.

Pleasure and Play

In some ways, pleasure is easier to define than mastery is, and it certainly is akin to play. But what we mean by pleasure is the felt sense of enjoyment or fun. This involves *hedonic* pleasure or a "sense" experience. As a rule, for pleasure to occur, there is no real objective or goal. If there is a goal to an activity, it probably is a mastery activity. Pleasant events are enjoyable not because of their outcomes, but because we get to engage in them. The number of pleasant events that people might describe is literally endless. They can range from looking at beautiful flowers, to eating a favorite food, to a relaxing in a hot bath, to engaging in hot sex. What these activities have in common is a kind of sensory input that the mind and body recognize and label as "good." That sensory input can be touch (e.g., massage), smell (e.g., flowers, perfume), sight (e.g., beautiful scenery), taste (e.g., food or drink), or sound (e.g., music, the sound of the sea).

Some pleasant activities engage a number of our senses, for example, swimming in a beautiful lake or the ocean touches us physically, looks beautiful, sounds pleasing, and smells refreshing when we reflect on the experience. Pleasure is also uniquely personal; not everyone enjoys the same things. A beach scene might appeal to those who enjoy hot sun, sand, and surf. Others may view that scene as too hot and sweaty, or too uncomfortable; they prefer a snowy setting. But this variety of opinions results in lots of choices and pleasures for your own specific needs, not anyone else's. Some pleasurable activities are fun to do with others, some are more enjoyable when done alone; in fact, solitary pleasures may be even more enjoyable because when we are alone we can soak up our experiences in a deeper way.

THE BALANCING ACT

When people are depressed, one of the markers of the illness is usually an imbalance between the areas of mastery and pleasure. Some depressed people have very few pleasurable experiences; they may turn to a kind of workaholism, filling their time with "productive" activities and events and leaving little room for anything else. Others may respond to being depressed by never really challenging themselves, sticking only to activities that are distracting or easy to do. Both ways of coping are not likely to lead to much improvement and may deepen the person's depression.

If there is a strong imbalance between the areas of mastery and pleasure, that is, between work and play, so that there are few activities you enjoy, your life can seem like endless drudgery, as if you are trudging on some kind of treadmill with no end in sight. Also, you don't get the benefit of being recharged by spending time on things you enjoy doing. In fact, people who work all the time are probably not all that efficient. In many cases, taking a break from work to do something distracting or pleasant actually can help you to refocus later on and to be more efficient. Physical activity, especially, pays huge dividends in terms of your ability to concentrate.

At another level, people who deny themselves pleasure frequently have issues about whether they are sufficiently deserving to have pleasures in their lives. Some describe a sense in which they must achieve something (a promotion, a raise in pay, or recognition) before they can allow themselves to feel "entitled" to enjoy themselves.

The problem with this kind of thinking is that, to a great extent, we need some pleasure in our lives to not be depressed. It is not something you can postpone. Moreover, everyone is entitled to some pleasures; enjoyment is a basic human right, not something that must be earned. I often "prescribe" pleasure as a way to help the depressed person take some initial steps to get out of the depression.

There are, however, some people who, once they've become depressed, must struggle to do anything except "fun" or "light" things. They may have been unable to work because of illness, and may now believe that by staying distracted they are giving themselves time and space to recover. The problem with this kind of imbalance is that overdoing pleasant activities can make them less potent; that is, the activities themselves may lose the ability to recharge the person. It may be much pleasanter to have an exquisite meal once a week than to have one every day. Also, such people may think that if they are "sick," they should rest or be very careful not to become overwhelmed. But their sense of self often suffers; they may begin to feel unable to tackle anything that presents even a small challenge. We all need some resistance to push against to feel okay with ourselves and to give us the confidence that we can handle challenges.

Furthermore, when people are occupied only with distractions, important matters start to pile up. The house may be neglected, financial affairs need attention, and deadlines may go by without being met. This, too, means that the distracting activities will lose some of their power to be enjoyable because all these other important matters weigh on your mind. For people in this situation, it is useful to think about what small, slightly challenging kinds of activities they might take on. Sometimes this could be doing chores around the home, such as cleaning, organizing, or making repairs, practical tasks related to the smooth running of their households that they have been delaying doing. Such tasks, coupled with some distractions and rewards, can set things right again. Also, doing them can raise people's self-confidence in their own problem-solving capabilities.

FIGURING OUT WHERE YOUR TIME GOES

The discussion above may ring a bell for you; there may be parts of those descriptions that you relate to. But to get a true sense of what needs to happen in your own life, you must get some kind of baseline of what you're doing right now, analyze that a bit, and then figure out what to add that could make a real difference.

Working with a Journal

You may recall from the introduction that we highly recommend buying a blank journal in order to work with the exercises that you will encounter while reading this book. We hope you acted on that recommendation, because you are now at the point where having such a journal to write in will be a valuable tool for getting the most benefit from the following material.

To figure out where your time goes, your first step should be to record what you really do with your time. One very useful way to do this is to take a blank page in your journal and create a weekly activity worksheet that will allow you to record what you do with all of your waking hours in an average week.

The way to do this is to draw a chart on a blank page in your journal with eight horizontal columns going across the page and seventeen rows going down the page. The vertical columns are for the days of the week and should be labeled from left to right. The first column, the one at the far left, is reserved for recording most of the hours of a day. Take a look at table 9.1 to see a model of what your chart should look like.

Table 9.1: Sample Weekly Activity Schedule

	Monday	Tuesday	Wednesday	Thursday	Friday	Saturday	Sunday
8:00 AM							
9:00 AM							
10:00 AM							
11:00 AM							
12:00 PM							
1:00 PM							
2:00 PM							
3:00 PM							
4:00 PM							
5:00 PM							
6:00 PM							
7:00 PM							
8:00 PM							
9:00 PM							
10:00 PM							
11:00 PM							
12:00 AM							

The idea is to fill in this chart for a week in order to record how you spend your time. To complete the worksheet, simply write a few words about what you do during each hour. Mostly, this will be one or two words (e.g., "working," "watching TV," "reading book," "at the gym," "with the kids"). It's fine to enter an activity once and then draw an arrow to indicate that the activity continues for whatever length of time is involved.

You will also want to rate your activities for how much (if any) pleasure and mastery they provide. The easiest way to do this is to rate each activity (not necessarily each hour, of course) from 0 to 10 for how much pleasure it gives you, with 10 as the most pleasant activity imaginable, and 0 as downright unpleasant.

Then, rate the level of mastery an activity gives you, again with 10 as the most mastery possible, and 0 being no mastery at all. For example, if you were to record your gardening activities it might look like this: "gardening," pleasure = 5, mastery = 7, whereas another record might be "having dinner out," pleasure = 7, mastery = 0. This suggests that gardening is mostly a mastery experience, but also enjoyable; whereas dinner out is enjoyable but doesn't lead to any particular sense of achievement.

WHAT YOUR SCHEDULE CAN TELL YOU

Once you've completed your worksheet, you'll use it to examine a number of areas, all with a view toward balancing your activities related to mastery and pleasure. The things to look for are these:

1. Overall, are your ratings for mastery or pleasure similar or are they quite different? Over the week, were there more "peaks" in the area of having fun or achieving goals? If you had more pleasure than mastery, consider challenging yourself a bit more and more often. If during the week you experienced more mastery than pleasure, consider adding some activities that would be enjoyable and give you something to look forward to.

2. Are there some activities that lead to a high mastery or pleasure rating (7 or more)? It will be important to have at least a handful of these events each week, activities that provide a kind of high point for the week in terms of either mastery or

pleasure. These are activities that have the potential to really give your self-confidence an important boost, or to give you something pleasant to look forward to.

3. Finally, would you recommend a similar routine to the people you love, your friends and family? In other words, do you believe that your routine would be beneficial for other people to follow? Do you think your routine has enough interesting things going on? That the amount of stress you deal with is "just right" (not overwhelming, but challenging)? Similarly, if this were the daily routine of your best friend, what suggestions would you make to him or her? Would you say "change nothing at all"? Or would you ask your friend to consider doing more mastery or pleasure activities? The approach of using "the best friend" perspective often leads to a considerable change in your own perspective on how you spend your time. You might want to say to your friend "take more time for yourself," or "get out there and try to accomplish some more things."

Once you've asked and answered these questions for yourself, you should have a better sense of what kinds of adjustments need to be made in your life to achieve better balance. Perhaps you can find a way to spend less time in activities that are neither very pleasant nor lead to a sense of mastery. This can be hard to do with certain things we "must" do (like work to earn money, or family responsibilities that we don't get much satisfaction from). However, many people are surprised to discover there are some activities they do purely out of habit. Activities that don't result in much satisfaction or fun. The important thing is to decide what to add to your daily routine. Do you need to spend more time with pleasant events and distractions? Are there enough meaningful challenges available to you?

ADDING ACTIVITIES

Once you have some sense of what you need to add to your weekly schedule, it's time to begin brainstorming activities you could try out. Looking at your options can be a fun, creative activity in itself. Feel free to draw on your past (things you used to do that were enjoyable), or your aspirations (I have always wanted to try _____ [fill in the blank]). Looking at your past can be important because, in a sense, you already know that these activities interested you at some time; they are known quantities. Looking at things you've always wanted to try, or dreamed of trying, taps into your personal aspirations.

Many of us have activities we'd like to try that we've put off for various reasons, mainly because we think we have plenty of time to get around to them, or we see some obstacle in the path that might make the activity difficult. One way to get ideas is to look around you and assess the ways that your friends and family enjoy themselves. This can be useful because you may already have a ready-made "buddy" to do fun things with.

For example, if you have a good friend who is an avid golfer, and you think you might enjoy golf, why not ask your friend to take you along on the next golfing outing, so you can check it out? Other places to think about are recreation centers, continuing education classes, fitness facilities, and community centers. All these places will have lots of announcements for future events and activities that might trigger a spark of interest in you. Also, there is the world of the Internet to explore. First, name any activity, hobby, pastime, sport, or indulgence. Then, type it into a search engine and you'll find hundreds of resources and interest groups.

TRYING THINGS OUT AND ASSESSING CHANGE

Once you've got some ideas about what you like to do, then it's time to sit down and plan what you'll do and when to start doing it. You are always more likely to succeed at trying out new activities when you plan carefully and pick a specific date and time to start. Remember, too, you don't want to end up feeling overwhelmed or stressed out; so, be sure to start any new activity in a gradual way. Sometimes, just to get started, you might first gather some information. If you want to learn how to paddle a canoe, you could start by looking at community recreation centers or, better yet, a shop that sells canoes. The personnel in such a shop may be able to tell you more about how to get going. Again, searching the Internet can be an enjoyable kind of activity in itself. For example, researching travel plans on the Internet can be an enjoyable pastime; it is after all a kind of travel of the mind.

Of course, not everything you plan will end up being as much fun or as satisfying as you hoped it would be. Remember that you can add any new activity to your weekly schedule as an experiment to see what, if any, difference it makes to your sense of mastery and your pleasure ratings. Just as you did with your "baseline" weekly activity schedule above, you can ask yourself the following questions to establish the value of new activity in your life:

1. What kind of mastery or pleasure rating do I give to the activity? (Remember, you are looking for levels of 7 or higher, whenever possible.)

2. Did something occur when I did the activity that I didn't expect? Was it better than I expected? You may discover that you enjoyed the activity more than you expected to. (Remember, depression really can undermine your ability to anticipate positive events, even when the event itself is positive.)

3. Were there any obstacles to doing the activity? What are the chances of being able to sustain the activity? Or was it more of a one-time only experience? (Remember, you are looking for an activity or activities that can become a regular part of your life, something that will provide you with an ongoing opportunity to enjoy yourself more often or something that will help you to feel better about your capabilities, talents, and skills.)

Your answers to these questions should help you to establish the value of whatever new activities you've begun to do.

MAINTAINING YOUR MOMENTUM

When using these strategies with depressed people, I've often found that there is some initial enthusiasm to do new things but that this enthusiasm can fade away much faster than I hoped it would. Sometimes, this happens after a few weeks of trying out a new behavior because, after people have made a real effort to change over several weeks, their old habits and routines can return and just obliterate their new activities.

Depressed people who have many obligations to meet are especially vulnerable to giving up on new pleasurable activities, often because they do begin to feel a little better when they start doing them. Then, because they feel better, they may begin to think they no longer need to schedule that pleasant event into their routine. That's why it's important to keep in mind that you've been asked to set only modest goals at first. Going to a movie, learning a hobby, going to a class may not be life-changing events. You may even end up thinking these activities are optional. But we hope that what results from this behavioral activation approach will be a profound shift in how you structure your life.

Your needs matter. The theme underlying these attempts at change is that your needs matter. No one can feel good or whole if they do not have time for themselves and do not engage in sufficiently satisfying work and play. People suffering from depression treat their own needs as expendable, and often view their obligations to other people as more important than their own needs. Eventually, that view of life will keep you from feeling well. Here's an analogy that makes this point in a very graphic way.

When traveling on a plane, we're always told what to do if the oxygen masks must be deployed. What should you do if the masks drop down and you are sitting next to someone who can't fasten his or her mask (e.g., a child, a disabled person)? Well, the instruction always tells you to fasten your mask first; then take care of the person beside you. It is not the other way around. Why not? Clearly, because putting the other person first puts you both at risk. If anything doesn't go perfectly, both you and the other person will not be able to breathe. By putting your own mask on first, you can literally survive long enough to be a real help to the person beside you. That's what your weekly routine should be like: first take good care of your body and spirit and only then share yourself with others and meet your obligations to them.

SLEEP FOR WELLNESS

Behavioral activation, which examines the ratio between the amount of time you spend on mastery and pleasure, clearly looks at your daily routine with a view toward giving you lots of options. But some parts of your daily routine should not be optional and cannot be left to chance.

Sleep is one of those areas, and this is especially true for someone with a physical or mental illness. Sleep provides one of the best ways to heal both the spirit and the mind. Good sleep is said to be "restorative," in that it restores us to a healthier, more energetic state when we awaken.

Sleep difficulties. One of the hallmarks of depression (and many other kinds of physical and emotional problems) is disturbed sleep or sleep that is "nonrestorative." People whose sleep is disturbed wake up and feel pretty much the way they did when they went to bed, or, they may feel even more tired than they did when they retired for the night. Psychologically, those people don't get a fresh start. Their brand-new day begins almost as though the day before has continued after a not very refreshing pause.

Research has demonstrated that sleep is a very important issue in depression. Disturbances in sleep patterns, either sleeping too much or too little, is a key symptom in diagnosing depression. In either case, the disturbed sleep usually results in feeling tired during the day. Some researchers believe that depression and sleep problems may share an ultimate cause, in fact, some researchers go so far as to describe depression as a sleep-related disorder (Ware and Morin 1997).

REM sleep. Mainly, depression seems to disrupt one particular stage of sleep, the REM stage. (*REM* stands for Rapid Eye Movement. This stage is the one in which we tend to dream.) Depressed people have less REM sleep and depressed people enter the REM stage of sleep more quickly than nondepressed people, possibly because their brain is trying to get more REM sleep in, but something else interferes with getting enough REM sleep over the course of the night (Rehm, Wagner, and Ivens-Tyndal 2001).

Another way in which we've learned how critical sleep can be to health and mood is by taking people who are otherwise well, and on an experimental basis only, depriving them of sleep and studying what happens. When people are deprived of REM sleep (this is done by very lightly "awakening" people so that they come out of REM, but don't actually wake up), the next day their behavior and emotions change, sometimes quite dramatically. The ability to cope with stress and frustration is the area most affected by REM deprivation. Sometimes, this is described as the person becoming "emotionally brittle," even though the subjects in these studies do go through all the other stages of sleep and they describe feeling rested after their sleep (Ware and Morin 1997).

So, it seems that REM sleep in particular helps us to sort through emotional thoughts and memories, which results in the ability to cope with new experiences. More generally, the better you sleep, the more likely you will be able to cope effectively with all kinds of illnesses, ranging from schizophrenia to cancer (Hofstetter, Lysaker, and Mayeda 2005).

Thyroid problems and sleep. The treatment for someone vulnerable to a biopsychosocial illness like those associated with thyroid problems is to do the best we can to improve the quality of the person's sleep. Sometimes this requires medication. If sleep is very disturbed and irregular, a sleep-aid medication may be indicated; your doctor can help you with this. Some of the prescription medication available for sleep disorders today is quite effective, and the newer formulations appear to help people wake up feeling refreshed. (In the past, most sleep medications made people feel groggy when they woke up, even after a full night of sleep.)

Side effects of sleep medication. However, even some of the best medications available are not without some costs and risks. Although these medications often are very effective in helping people to fall asleep and stay asleep, there are common side effects. One is that, over time, more medication may be needed to achieve the same results. Also, once the medication is stopped, there can be a "rebound" effect in which, because your body has become used to the medication, trying to fall asleep without it is harder than it might have been when you first started taking it. This is why it's important to talk to your doctor about any sleep problems you may be having. If your sleep is very poor, using medications may help you get restarted on good, restful sleep. That might make the side effects and the rebound worthwhile. Luckily, however, there are also some easy things that you can try that have no side effects that can make a huge difference to your sleep quality.

SLEEP HYGIENE: MAXIMIZE YOUR CHANCES OF A GOOD NIGHT'S REST

The first step in getting a good night's sleep is to leave yourself enough time for it. The weekly schedule you created earlier in this chapter to figure out where you spend your time can come in handy for this. As I said, the first step toward sleeping better is to make sure that you allow enough time in your schedule for sleep. Most people need about eight hours of sleep (give or take an hour). So, that means if you go to bed at 11 PM, you should not rise before 7 AM. Your time to sleep should be "protected time," and, as much as possible, have no trespasses from your late night activities or very early morning obligations. This seems like such a basic maxim, but it is very much at risk in our culture of late-night television, early-bird news and business tickers, and the North American desire to pack the most we can into one day.

Dr. Stanley Coren has made a compelling case that Western culture has turned sleep into a dispensable activity. He describes many of the societal factors that have made inroads on our need (and right) for sleeping time, including such changes as daylight savings time (which seems to result in more car accidents), shift work, and a trend in which the need for sleep is seen by some as a moral or personal failing (Coren 1996). This couldn't be more at odds with the scientific data that tell us just how critical a good night's sleep really is.

In addition to protecting your time devoted to sleeping, good sleep hygiene incorporates a number of rules and suggestions that are described below (Bootzin and Rider 1997):

1. **Go to bed at the same time every night and get up at the same time every morning.** This is the best way to train the internal clock of your body as to when it is time to be awake and when it is time to be asleep. Whenever possible, avoid the temptation to sleep in on weekend mornings or to stay up late on weekends nights. At first, keeping a record of sleep and wake times may be hard. You may not want to go to bed when you should, or you feel like hitting the snooze button in the morning when you should be awake. But try it. Eventually, you might find that you will become tired just when you expect to, and that you awaken without the need for an alarm clock. It's a simple strategy, but it can be very effective.

2. **Avoid alcohol and caffeine.** It's easy to fall into the habit of using caffeinated drinks to "wake up" in the morning and having an alcoholic nightcap before going to bed. These habits should be avoided as much as possible; at the very least, don't consume either substance within four hours of trying to go to sleep or of awakening. Both caffeine and alcohol have subtle addictive properties, even in small quantities,

when it comes to sleep. People can become reliant on them fairly quickly and may need more and more over time to get the desired effect. Moreover, these substances certainly don't help you to fall asleep naturally.

3. **Beds are for sleeping.** "Beds are for sleeping" is a catch-phrase for the idea that you should do nothing else in your bed but sleep. You never want your bed to become associated with other activities like eating, watching television, doing work, or, worst of all, worrying and insomnia. When you retire to bed, give yourself ten minutes to fall asleep. If that doesn't work, don't stay in bed. If you do, you risk associating being in bed and struggling to fall asleep. Instead, get up and try something distracting, something to occupy your mind. Try something as simple as getting up, moving to a chair, and reading a book. Then, if you do start to get noticeably tired again, you can try falling asleep in your bed again. Too many people when trying to fall sleep or when they wake up at the wrong time, stay in bed. Often they worry and wrack their brains about their lack of sleep. And, of course, trying so hard to fall asleep is the opposite of what your mind needs to be doing to get to sleep! You want to be sure that your bed doesn't become your place to worry. When that happens, the act of going to bed will often initiate a cycle of worry and rumination.

4. **Slow down well before going to bed.** Your body and mind need time to wind down after being awake and busy. For that reason it's important not to be too busy or too physically stimulated before bedtime. It can be very difficult for your body and mind to go from a fast pace to the slow pace of sleep in a few minutes or even an hour. Some people experience problems with this when they work late into the evening and go to bed immediately after arriving home. Often, they are still "revved up" and may need two to three hours of downtime before they can sleep. Strong emotions can also create sleep difficulties, so if you know that you must have a difficult conversation or do something that stirs up strong emotions, try to do it well before you retire. As a rule, don't do any exercise or any challenging activity two hours before retiring if that is possible.

5. **Make your sleeping environment comfortable.** Remember that your sleeping environment should be as comfortable as possible. Make sure your bed is comfortable and supportive. It is often surprising how long people will use a mattress that isn't ideal for them. Somehow, the bed seems to be last in line for replacement or maintenance. These days there are so many choices regarding mattress types that the chances are good you will find something you like much better than what you currently have. Also, mattresses need some care. Some need to be turned over periodically, and they do wear with time and use.

   The degree of darkness is another issue that is often overlooked. Some people use bedroom curtains that aren't able to keep out enough light. Sound is important too. Make sure that your environment is as quiet and undisturbed as possible; it is not wise to sacrifice your own sleep because of a pet (or child) who wants to sleep in your bed with you, but wakes you every hour. The bottom line is to avoid making compromises about what is comfortable for you. Sleep really is that precious.

6. **No napping.** This is the most straightforward rule of sleep hygiene, but it is also quite difficult to follow when your sleep has been disrupted. Naps tend to make it hard to fall asleep later, although your body can work hard to convince you that you need to sleep "right now!" The fact is, a nap, especially if it's longer than twenty minutes, does begin to reset your body clock. It's a bit like traveling across time zones and getting jet lag; naps can throw off the internal timekeeping your body does, and they may make it difficult to fall asleep when you want to or need to get some sleep.

EXERCISE

Regular exercise is another activity that, like sleep, should not be left to chance. Exercise can be a potent source of mastery and pleasure. For some, a workout, jog, or walk is a real pleasure. For others, these activities don't evoke even an ounce of pleasure, but doing them would certainly be an achievement. Exercise has so many positive physical benefits that looking at it only through the lens of mastery and pleasure is inadequate. Exercise is one of the few things in life that has no downside. It is nothing but upside.

What Exercise Can Do for You

The physical benefits of exercise for our bodies and medical health are obvious. There isn't a single health organization that doesn't recommend exercise as part of its standard practice. In fact, most medical groups (ranging from the American Medical Association to the World Health Organization) have people and programs that try to address the gap between the recommendations they make, and what actually happens out there in the real world. Even for healthy people, getting enough regular exercise is a hard-to-solve challenge. Wishing that people would exercise more won't make it so. It's very important for you to understand the reasons why exercise would be beneficial for you.

The fact is, we already have studies that prove to us that depression responds well to exercise. For example, in one study, depressed people were randomly assigned to enroll in a moderate exercise program, take placebos (sugar pills), or get no treatment at all. It turned out that the exercise program changed symptoms more than a placebo or no treatment; this was especially true in cases of mild and moderate depression (Tkachuk and Martin 1999). Another study examined different kinds of exercise intensity, including an exercise placebo (simple stretching), again in people with mild to moderate depression. These researchers found that a moderate level of exercise reduced depression scores by almost 50 percent on average (Dunn et al. 2005). Overall, it seems that exercise is particularly effective when depression starts to lift, and when it is used as an adjunct to other treatments, including antidepressants (Brosse et al. 2002).

How Much Exercise Do You Need?

One of surprising things about the connection between exercise and depression is that you don't need to run marathons or become a bodybuilder to get the desired effects. Three times a week of moderate exercise (brisk walking, slow jogging, cycling at a medium pace) for about thirty minutes or more is sufficient to benefit your mood. It doesn't seem to matter much whether this level of exercise is spread over three or five days; what matters is the overall level of energy that is expended (Dunn et al. 2005).

Exactly why exercise is so helpful is still hard to say; we don't fully understand how it works as well as we should. So far, we know that exercise has many positive effects on the brain; it results in having more of the chemicals that help to build and maintain neurons, it protects the brain from injury, and it improves learning and memory (Cotman and Berchtold 2002). At the same time, people who exercise also experience increases in self-worth, and there's no doubt that exercise is a potent source of mastery. Again, it's important to remember that the mind and body are part of the same "whole" and one always affects the other. People who exercise vigorously will tell you that whatever their mental state is prior to a workout, once they've completed the workout, they are in a different, better frame of mind.

You've probably heard of "runner's high," which does seem to be caused by changes in the neurotransmitters that result from exercise. Most of us will experience something like runner's high after moderate exercise. So, to try to become more motivated to exercise, remember what exercise will do for you in the short term, and that the long-term reward in terms of years of healthy living is incalculable.

Getting Started on an Exercise Program

Before starting any new exercise plan, take the time to check in with your doctor. Most likely, he or she will be more than encouraging, but there are some things that must be looked at before you begin. Once you've got your doctor's okay, try the following:

1. **Keep it simple.** Start with something that has a relatively low entry cost; if you want to exercise by windsurfing, it's going to be a lot more work than if you want to walk or jog. The chances of sticking to an exercise routine go way up when it is readily available to you. What could be easier than buying a pair of good running shoes and running in a park or on paved sidewalks? Sometimes people invest in expensive gym memberships or equipment (shown on late-night TV) that ends up collecting dust because most people find that things done on impulse do not last. Ease your way into the new activity, and before you commit your money and time, make sure it's for you.

2. **Start small.** If you have been sedentary or not exercising at all, your first day out don't do any more than walk one block. Don't try to get to an aerobic, out-of-breath level your first day, or even your second. Add additional time or distance to your exercise very gradually. Some people are tempted to throw themselves into a new routine right away, like jogging six miles on their first day out. Chances are, if you did this, you'd be sore the next day, and maybe even collect an injury. That exercise session could become a traumatic memory you are not eager to repeat.

   On the other hand, if you jogged for eight minutes your first day out, and added another four minutes a day, until you reached fifty to sixty minutes, in four weeks you might be jogging about six miles a day. And you would have become more comfortable with that distance gradually, had less chance of injuring yourself, and made the whole exercise commitment much more manageable.

3. **Find an exercise buddy.** Probably many other people in your life are also interested in exercising and may be struggling to find the time or to establish a routine. If you can identify these people and ask them to join you, you will have a much better chance of maintaining your exercise plan over the long run. Knowing that someone else is counting on you to show up may motivate you on those days you don't feel like exercising. Working out with a buddy also makes a more public commitment to exercising regularly, which will help you stay on track. Also, it doesn't hurt that, along with your exercise, you'll have a social aspect to your workout. A jog always goes by faster when there is also an interesting conversation on the trot.

4. **Make exercise "work" for you.** One way to make exercise a part of your daily routine is to make it serve a purpose for you. One great example, if it's possible, would be walking to work. Although it might take you longer than driving or taking public transportation, it might be easier to add into your routine since getting to work is already likely to be a part of your life. Also, when you are at work, or out anywhere in the world, using the stairs instead of taking elevators is a great way to add exercise into your day without adding much time.

5. **Make it fun to do.** In the same way that people are attracted to different sensations and feelings, they also have different types of affinities for exercise. If you are someone who loves music and dance, an aerobics class that programs movements to music might be just the ticket. If you enjoy the sensation of speed, cycling could be your kind of workout. If you like contemplating nature, hiking might be your thing. If you're the sort of person who enjoys socializing, weight training at a gym might be just right. (There's always lots of time between sets.) Again, we are far more likely to continue with exercise routines that have some kind of hedonic pleasure attached to them. Here, the end may justify the means.

6. **Pick a time, any time.** Perhaps more than planning any other activity, to get into a regular exercise schedule, it's important to plan exactly when and where. This maximizes the likelihood that you won't make excuses or rationalizations to get out of doing it. Most exercise does involve some preparation; even walking briskly will require sturdy walking shoes and comfortable clothing. If you don't plan properly, you may sabotage yourself by not having the gear you need when you need it.

We surely understand that establishing an exercise routine is a tall order for most of you. As with any new healthy behavior, your exercise progress may go by fits and starts. Many of us have histories of expensive gym memberships that went unused, exercise bicycles used as clothes hangers, and weight-training equipment collecting dust under the couch. The trick is to keep trying different forms of exercise until you find the one that works for you. Your overall goal, after all, is to put more of your energy into exercise this week than last week, from one month to the next, one year to the next. Physical exercise needs to become a part of your lifestyle.

MEANING AND SPIRITUALITY

At first, it may seem odd to discuss behavioral activation, sleep, exercise, and then segue into spiritual matters. And yet they are related. Increasingly, psychologists have been dealing with these issues because they do appear to be so critical to a sense of wellness. Concepts such as core values have become a focus for experts on behavioral change (Hayes, Strosahl, and Wilson 1999). These clinicians believe that we must look beyond a simple balance between mastery and pleasurable activities, although achieving this balance is a critical building block to better mental health.

But to achieve true wellness and a high quality of life it is also important that what we do each day reflects our values. We need to believe our actions serve a purpose we understand as more important than we are. So, I am not, strictly speaking, talking about religion. Values can be abstract concepts like the duty to be charitable or to protect human rights, which are also aspects of some religious philosophies, but may be a part of humanistic and other philosophic disciplines, too. Moreover, there is plenty of data from researchers that supports the value of spiritual practices for health.

Researchers have found that patients suffering from neurological disorders, heart disease, renal failure, AIDS, and other physical disorders who practice a spiritual discipline feel more in control of their difficulties and their lives, and have lower levels of stress and distress (Koenig, Larson, and Larson 2001). Having a purpose in life seems to help with depression too (Braam et al. 2001). The positive impact of spirituality on depression is not due to religious observance per se; for example, people who observe religious practices out of a sense of obligation or who are externally pressured to do so are actually at risk of depression (Murphy et al. 2000). But religious activities that come from within the person, that the person really believes in doing, actually seem to protect him or her from depression even when the practitioner does not attend religious services regularly.

The whole notion of meaning, and its importance to health, entered psychology only after the second World War, thanks to the work of Viktor Frankl. Frankl spent most of the war years in a concentration camp, which brought him face to face with his and others' mortality every day. He secretly kept notes of his time as a prisoner, which he developed into his gripping book *Man's Search for Meaning* (1959) after the war. It is difficult to summarize this great book. But Frankl's thesis holds that maintaining a sense of meaning was, literally, critical for survival in the camps, not only psychologically, but also physically, as well.

Those fellow prisoners who gave up all of their beliefs, who believed in nothing, were at much higher risk of being killed, or dying of other causes. Frankl maintained throughout his experience that a person could *choose* to find meaning, even in the midst of such great suffering.

At first, Frankl tried to find meaning for his life in his love for his wife, and through this he came to appreciate even tiny fragments of beauty in his surroundings or in glimpses of humanity among his cap-tors. Later, he came to see himself as more of a leader; he recognized that his real purpose in life was to try to help others to not give up and to keep hope alive. Eventually, Frankl's work resulted in a form of treatment called *logotherapy* in which the focus is to look for and find the meaning of one's experiences, particularly suffering.

So, we highly recommend giving some thought to this very pri-vate, and very important, part of your daily life. And we encourage you to take action around the meaning of your life and the values you want to share with the world. For some, this might mean rediscovering their religious roots and reestablishing regular contact with a congregation or ministry. For others, this might trigger more of a philosophical quest to find a discipline that works for them that they have not yet consid-ered. Whether it be Buddhist meditation, Catholic Mass, or serving food at a homeless shelter, what we ask you to do is to consider taking some action around a spiritual discipline or meaning-of-life practice.

One good place to start would be to ask yourself this question: "Is there a reason I get out of bed that is more important than I and my immediate needs are?" This is not to suggest that your needs aren't important or that they shouldn't be a priority. But what the question really tries to get at is whether there is something larger that you believe in, something more important than the fact that you are tired and depressed. Whatever it is that you get out of bed for is probably part of the meaning of your life. Focusing on and enhancing that will add a great deal to the quality and stability in your life.

Summary

In this chapter we've considered a great many lifestyle factors and how they relate to your positive mental and physical health. Balance has been the key theme; the balance between activity and rest, mastery and pleasure, fun and work. These elements need to be in harmony for a high quality of life. We've asked you to think about the changes you might make to lead a better life; whether they might be in having more fun, getting more restful sleep, or adding a spiritual practice to your daily routines.

Each small change you make in these areas will pay big dividends over time. Don't be fooled by how simple these actions appear to be; I've never worked with anyone who regretted becoming more active and more vitally involved, or who didn't feel better by choosing his or her activities more wisely. But we also know that maintaining what seem like small changes is hard. People can backslide very quickly into a stressed-out or daily routine that just isn't as involving as it needs to be when they aren't careful. So it's worth keeping your eye on the ball of your daily routines, and making sure you are getting the most you can out of every day.

CHAPTER 10

Cognitive Strategies

In chapter 8, I described the very intimate connection between the mind and the body. This connection has two components: the body affects the mind, but the mind also affects the body. Often, the second part is less obvious. Most of us understand that when we exercise, eat in a healthy and balanced way, and get sufficient amounts of restful sleep, our mental state will be clearer, more focused, even-tempered, and more relaxed compared to how we are when we neglect some of these physical aspects of living. In fact, when we talk about the mind-body connection, quite often this is what most people mean. But those physical aspects are only half of the equation; the mind-body connection is a two-way street.

The mind also affects the body. Mental events, mental habits, and the way we think and feel affect how well our body systems function. Events in the mind are often played out in our bodies, sometimes beneath the level of our awareness. If you have any doubts about this, consider the following two examples that may make this connection clearer.

FEAR AND THE FIGHT-OR-FLIGHT SYNDROME

First, let's consider the matter of fear, which is a universal human response when we are threatened in some way, or more importantly, when we *believe* we are threatened or that danger is imminent. Flying in an airplane provides a situation that can give us pause. Imagine you are sitting in a plane cruising along above the clouds. You're comfortably seated, watching the in-flight movie, and eating the ever-present peanuts. If you were asked just then to describe your physical state or if your body could be scanned in some way, we might find that your physical state is fairly normal, even relaxed.

Now imagine that you hear a loud bang coming from deep inside the plane's engines, followed by a violent shaking and pitching in the passenger cabin. What would we see if we scanned your body now? We'd see a classic picture of the *fight-or-flight syndrome*. A *syndrome* is a collection of symptoms. In this syndrome, the sympathetic nervous system ramps up, and the heart rate increases dramatically, blood flow to the muscles and extremities of the body increases, skin temperature rises, and a host of other physiological changes take place. This would be a normal fear reaction, triggered not by any real physical malfunction, but by your mind perceiving a danger and causing your body to react. Your mind tells your body "I see danger coming," and makes sure that the right chemical messengers are transmitted to your body to activate the fight-or-flight syndrome, otherwise known as the fear response.

Now, consider a second example, perhaps trivial, but an interesting demonstration of the mind's ability to affect the body. Imagine you are having dinner in a nice restaurant when, in plain sight, a diner at another table slumps into his chair, then keels over and vomits onto the floor. Kind of a disgusting thought, right? What tends to happen in a situation like this is that people who witness the event also begin to feel nauseous. One moment they are delighting in their filet mignon and shrimp scampi, the next minute they are pushing their plates away and wondering whether to walk or run to the bathroom. Even reading about a scenario like this might trigger some amount of nausea or queasiness. How can this be?

Well, it seems that this syndrome is an evolutionary response designed to protect us. Sudden, violent vomiting can be a sign of spoiled food; it's the body's way of trying to get rid of a noxious substance as quickly as possible. In primitive societies and among groups of animals where food is shared, seeing a peer vomit while eating appears to be a cue that says something like, "If this food is causing that person to become sick, then there must be something wrong with the food I am eating too. Better safe than sorry. I'll tell my body to vomit." So, although it may seem controversial to say that you can think your way into vomiting, it is literally true in these kinds of circumstances.

So, where are we headed with this idea that your mind and the body are so intimately connected in terms of cause and effect? Well, the logical good news holds that if we can do things to change the way we perceive a situation, then we can change the way we feel, and literally change our biology. You may think this is a little extreme, but today there is a vast amount of data that suggests that people who learn how to use "self-talk" in psychotherapy and who practice particular skills involving their thoughts can alter the way their brain works, and even the way their thyroid gland functions. So it's important to look at this area in some detail.

COGNITIVE BEHAVIORAL THERAPY

The specific kind of self-talk under discussion here is called *cognitive behavioral therapy* (CBT). This type of psychotherapy was first developed in the 1960s to deal with depression. I will describe a bit about what it is and how it works, and then I'll describe how the skills taught in CBT are especially useful for people with thyroid problems.

Back in the 1960s, Dr. Aaron T. Beck was particularly interested in depression, and over the course of the following decades he developed CBT. The key advance Dr. Beck made occurred when he began to ask his patients direct questions about the content of their thoughts. This was quite controversial at that time because the standard approach to treating depression then was psychoanalysis, Sigmund Freud's method. Psychoanalysis involves the patient doing almost all of the talking and the therapist making relatively few interpretations based on what the patient says.

Beck stepped out of this passive role and used different research methods to question his patients about their depression and other experiences. His patients described to him a *stream of consciousness*—a flow of words or self-talk—that was going on just below the surface of their everyday conversation. For some people, their flow of self-talk was like an audiotape that never stopped playing. It was like a continuous murmur (or mutter) that accompanied most thoughts and conversations his patients experienced. Moreover, this stream of consciousness was very negative in its tone.

Dr. Beck found that depressed people were having an internal conversation with themselves that was frequently pessimistic, hopeless, and much more negative than was realistic. It was as if depressed people were wearing eyeglasses that filtered out all the positive information from their environment and focused only on negative assessments of themselves (Beck 1967; Clark, Beck, and Alford 1999).

The idea that thoughts influence negative feelings is often referred to as the *cognitive* or *cognitive behavioral approach* to understanding depression. The word *cognitive* just means "thinking" or "mental processing." When we feel well, our internal thoughts or cognitions tend to be either positive or neutral. However, as stated earlier, Beck's critically important observation was that people who are depressed interpret many of their circumstances as negative, even when their negative views are unrealistic; that is, these negative views do not correspond to how things really are.

It's very important to say here that this doesn't necessarily mean that negative thinking triggers depression. Instead, this approach says that depression is accompanied by negative thinking. So, regardless of whether depression is triggered by a biological problem or not, negative thinking will be an important part of the depressed person's problem. Once negative thinking gets started, it can become very difficult to control because it feeds on itself in what is sometimes called a negative spiral. Once a depression gets started, for whatever reason, it tends to continue on its own unless the whole problem is examined from the critically important biopsychosocial approach (see chapter 8 for a discussion on this approach).

THE THYROID, DEPRESSION, AND CBT

When depression is the result of a thyroid problem, we know that getting the thyroid to function properly by using and fine-tuning medications is fundamental, without which it is very difficult to fully recover. But as I've said elsewhere, fixing only the biology may not cure the whole problem. Using the strategies of CBT will add a useful tool. We know from over twenty years of careful research that CBT is a very effective treatment for depression and has a lot of research support (Clark, Beck, and Alford 1999). This research tells us that CBT is as effective for treating depression as antidepressant medication and that it works well in the long run in that it can prevent relapses if the skills of CBT continue to be practiced (Bieling and Antony 2003; Rowa, Bieling, and Segal, forthcoming).

There is even more interesting research that has been developed in the last few years, some of it critical for those with thyroid problems. First, researchers have begun to explore how CBT works by studying the brains of those people who are being treated. One of the most important recent studies compared the brains of people being treated with cognitive therapy for sixteen sessions and others being treated for the equivalent length of time with Paxil, a well-known antidepressant (Goldapple et al. 2004).

All of the people in the study had brain scans using *positron emission tomography* (PET). PET works by injecting small amounts of radioactive chemicals into the body that make their way to the brain. Inside a PET scanner, the radioactive chemicals become part of the brain's activity; they are attracted to places where the brain is doing its metabolic work and tend to not be present in places where the brain is relatively inactive. A scanner can reveal where the radioactivity, and hence activity, is in the brain and translates the activity into different colors. You can think of it as similar to the radar maps we often see, where bright spots mean more rain or weather activity. The brighter the area, the more chemicals are present and hence the greater the level of activity; all of this allows researchers to see exactly how the brain is operating at a given point.

In this study, each participant had two separate brain scans, one before treatment started, and one when treatment ended. The researchers discovered a remarkable finding, one they did not expect. First, they noted distinct changes in the subjects' brains from the time the depressed people began treatment to the time they had recovered from depression, either by using CBT or the antidepressant, Paxil (Goldapple et al. 2004). Second, the kinds of brain changes they found differed, depending on which treatment people they had received.

In other words, both Paxil and CBT changed brain function but in very distinctive ways. CBT increased activity levels near the front of the brain, the part that governs thought. Paxil decreased activity in an area known as the hippocampus.

In a sense then, the researchers believed that CBT had changed symptoms by increasing people's ability to critically analyze their thoughts. For many people, this study and others like it have been eye-openers. Although it's obvious that the medications that change neurotransmitter levels also change brain chemistry and function, it is amazing that several weeks of talk therapy also change the brain. The conclusion seems to be this: Just as we know that biology affects psychology, so, too, does psychology affect biology.

From the perspective of thyroid function, another study is even more important. In this study, participants had their thyroid hormones checked before and after treatment with CBT (Joffe, Segal, and Singer 1996). The people in this study got twenty sessions of cognitive therapy. Those participants who improved during the CBT treatment showed decreases in their levels of the thyroid hormone T4; those who did not improve showed increases in their levels of the T4 hormone.

To sum up, CBT offers an effective way to treat depression and it is a way to connect mind and body. CBT offers a treatment that goes beyond antidepressant medication, in part, because it is a skill you can learn and use, like developing a healthy habit. What follows are ways to learn and use this approach.

WAYS TO CHANGE YOUR THINKING

There are two ways to become good at CBT. The first is to seek out a cognitive behavioral therapist and begin to work with that person. It's likely this will involve an investment of some of your time and financial resources. The second way to learn CBT strategies is to use a self-help approach.

Working with a therapist. CBT is usually a short-term treatment; most of the skills can be learned in about twenty sessions. However, your therapist will ask you to practice the skills you learn between sessions at home, as well as in the therapist's office.

When trying to find a therapist, there are several factors to consider. If you are seeking CBT, be sure to check out the therapist's credentials. One way to do this is to check out the listings of the Academy of Cognitive Therapy (ACT; www.academyofct.org) whose members have all been carefully screened for their expertise in practicing this kind of treatment. Also, the Association for Behavior and Cognitive Therapies (ABCT; www.aabt.org) can provide excellent referrals to practitioners who identify themselves as CBT practitioners, although unlike ACT, ABCT does not thoroughly verify the credentials of its members.

Once you find a therapist, it will be important that you trust the therapist, that you view the therapist as empathic, and that you believe that you and the therapist are working toward the same goal. Remember, you are the client who is buying a service; therefore, if you feel that the therapist is not a good fit with you, you should exercise your right of choice.

However, we recommend that you give a therapist with good credentials a solid try, say, three or four sessions, before you make a final decision about whether the relationship with the therapist can be productive.

Using a self-help approach. A self-help approach is the other way to learn CBT strategies. For example, Dennis Greenberger and Christine Padesky (1995) wrote an excellent book entitled *Mind Over Mood* that takes the reader, step by step, through the strategies that can help to change depressed thinking. Another good resource is a book by David Burns (1999), *The Feeling Good Handbook*. It describes exercises specifically related to thinking and depression. I will describe some of these skills in the rest of this chapter to get you started.

GETTING HOLD OF YOUR THOUGHTS

There are several steps to becoming able to grapple with your thoughts and emotions. The basic process can be summarized in four steps. I call the first step "getting hold of your thoughts," which means becoming aware of your self-talk. We all carry on an internal dialogue—a stream of consciousness, if you will—that goes on more or less constantly. This is a stream of thoughts that may have something to do with what we are currently doing but, at other times, it is preoccupied with something else.

Some activities receive our full attention, that is, our focused concentration. For example, balancing your checkbook or playing a skillful game like tennis or golf might receive all of your focused concentration. But think back to the last time you were at a social event and were bored, or you found yourself watching a dull television program. At those times, your mind quickly took you elsewhere.

For example, while bored at a party, you might have ended up thinking about other things you could be doing, even when you were conversing with other people at the event. While watching TV, slightly bored, you might have recalled you had bills you needed to pay. Or you might have had a thought about a work assignment. Such internal dialogue may have influenced your behavior, so that if you remembered you had outstanding bills, you might have ended up going to look for them.

Our internal dialogues are rarely turned off. Most of the time they give us helpful cues (like reminding us of unpaid bills). But this dialogue, which we take as a given and rarely notice, also can cause us a lot of grief. What if that interior voice was giving us unhelpful advice and we didn't know it? And that's precisely where the trouble starts: our self-talk is such a part of us that we experience it as "me," and most of the time we listen to it without questioning it. That's why when we are depressed, our thoughts are so important and so subversive. So, starting to become aware of your internal dialogue is step number one in this process.

The Mood Shift

Trying to track down your thoughts all the time would be very challenging and, most likely, impossible. But tracking all your thoughts all the time isn't necessary for CBT, because what we are interested in here are particular kinds of thoughts, that is, negative thoughts or automatic thoughts. Oddly enough, the way to delve into your thoughts is to pay attention to your *mood*. Remember, depression and thinking are connected. So, if you can notice your mood changing, you can often detect a change in your thinking as well.

In CBT, changes in mood are called *mood shifts*, which are exactly what they sound like, moments when you notice that your mood has shifted from one state to another. Because we are discussing depression, in this instance, we look for mood changes during which you begin feeling worse, perhaps sadder, more upset, tense, nervous, or more hopeless. Often this happens when certain events take place. Perhaps you get some bad news or an awful event happens. Life can be full of frustrations and little disappointments: a promotion you expected, but didn't get; a disagreement you had in an important relationship; other people letting you down; getting negative feedback from your boss; losing something important to you, or, worst of all, someone you love. All of these things happen as part of the human condition. But in a depression, they feel ever so much more powerful and long-lasting, and they do so in large part because of our thoughts.

So, to get a grip on your thoughts, even to get what you are thinking down on paper, you first need to practice paying attention to the shifts in your mood. At first, this might not seem difficult, but some people find it easier to do than others. Sometimes, a mood shift seems to come out of the blue, because nothing appears to have happened. And yet, looking at it again, often this shift took place because the person had a negative thought. When you've just received sad or bad news, it's usually pretty easy to relate the event to your mood. In CBT, we use a special diary we call a "thought worksheet" to facilitate understanding the relationship between events and low mood.

Monitoring Your Moods and Thoughts

To understand how to do this, you will need to open your journal to two blank facing pages, and then copy the sample thought worksheet form from table 10.1 below to the blank page on the left-hand side of your journal. Do not write anything on the right-hand page, because you will need to write on it to complete this exercise later in this chapter.

You'll notice that the sample form has three columns labeled Situation, Emotions, and Thoughts. The copy you create in your journal should also have three columns with the same three headings. Be sure to leave some room under the headings for some additional text that will help you to understand what to record.

Under Situation, write "Record what was happening when my mood shifted. What was going on? Was anyone else involved? Where was I?"

Under Emotions, write "What was I feeling? What are the words to describe what I was feeling?"

Under Thoughts, write "What was going through my mind just then? What was I saying to myself?" Be sure you leave plenty of space under each heading to record information in each column.

Situation. Now, let's start with a simple example. Think about the last time you were very sad or upset. Perhaps you received some bad news about a family member, or you got some negative feedback from your boss. Perhaps you quarreled with a loved one. When you've decided on the situation that you'd like to work on, write a brief description of it in the column under Situation. Try to keep your description as brief as you can. Sum it up in two or three sentences at the most.

For example, a client of mine, Kelly, the mother of a four-year-old daughter, got into a nasty argument with her husband. Her daughter

Table 10.1: Thought Worksheet

Situation	Emotions	Thoughts
Record what was happening when my mood shifted. What was going on? Was anyone else involved? Where was I?	What was I feeling? What are the words to describe what I was feeling?	What was going through my mind just then? What was I saying to myself?

Table 10.1: Sample Thought Worksheet

Situation	Emotions	Thoughts
Record what was happening when my mood shifted. What was going on? Was anyone else involved? Where was I?	What was I feeling? What are the words to describe what I was feeling?	What was going through my mind just then? What was I saying to myself?
Playing with Katie outside, John came over when Katie skinned her knee and got upset.	*Sad* *Hurt* *Angry*	*How could he say that to me?* *I was watching her closely.* *This could have happened if he was watching her.* *Why is it always up to me to watch Katie?* *He thinks I'm a bad mother.*

had fallen down in the yard and was crying because of a small scrape on her knee. Her husband came out of the house and questioned Kelly about what happened. At one point he said to her in an angry voice, "Why weren't you watching her?" So, under Situation, Kelly wrote, "Playing with Katie outside. John came out when Katie skinned her knee and got upset with me."

Emotions. Next, think about the emotions you felt during your situation. In our sample, under Emotions, Kelly wrote "sad," "hurt," and "angry." Notice that each of her entries in the Emotions column consists of one word. That's important because, almost always, emotions can be described with just a single word.

However, one situation can trigger several different emotions. Kelly was clearly hurt by John's accusation, but at the same time, she was also angry with him. You can expect some situations to involve several complicated emotions, some of which may even contradict each other.

As you try your hand at recording a situation that shifted your mood, you may want to ask yourself: "When did the shift occur? What time of day was it, what was going on, and who was around?" Often, recording the situation is relatively easy because something definitely happened to you; at times, however, the situation may be subtle and it may be hard to identify what triggered your negative mood. In fact, sometimes, there isn't much of a triggering event at all; instead, something really minor happens that triggers a negative thought, and it's actually the negative thought that triggers the emotions.

When it comes to writing down your emotions, sometimes it helps to write down your physical feelings, especially if those feelings relate to fear or dread. Emotions do affect us physically. They take place in the body as much as in the mind, and, sometimes, the way we feel physically affects our emotions. Basically, though, there are no right or wrong responses when you work with a thought worksheet. Eventually, you'll find the process of describing your emotions becoming easier and quicker.

Thoughts. Now comes the slightly harder part. We are used to dealing with the idea that an event or situation can cause us to feel something, that is, to react emotionally to the event or situation. In fact, though, our thoughts come in between the situation and the emotion. The thoughts occur in the middle of the process, like the meat in a sandwich. Learning to recognize your thoughts, however fleeting they may be, is the challenge. That's what this exercise is all about.

At first, this will take a while. For example, in Kelly's case, under Thoughts she wrote several—all of which were associated with different emotions—including "How could he say that to me?" "I was watching her closely." "This could have happened if he was watching her." "Why is it always up to me to watch Katie?" And she ended by writing, "He thinks I'm a bad mother."

So, you can see that Kelly wrote down her stream of consciousness; that is, what she said to herself when her husband spoke to her so angrily. To try this out with your own situation, ask yourself questions like these:

- What was I saying to myself?

- What thoughts went through my mind?

- What was I telling myself?

At the beginning, it may take you anywhere from a few minutes to half an hour to complete the blank page in your journal. The more you practice, though, the faster you'll become.

Thoughts are not full sentences. Remember, too, that your internal dialogue or automatic thoughts are not necessarily completely formed sentences. They may be more like quick talking points, short notes to yourself. Note that these kinds of emotional thoughts often occur very quickly, may seem beyond your conscious control, and are often biased or extremist in some way. In contrast, rational or intellectual thoughts require a lot more effort, are slow in coming, and tend not to have very much emotion attached to them. For most of us, there is something very personal, perhaps even embarrassing, about writing down these fleeting and often painful innermost thoughts. You may write down a thought and then find yourself thinking "that's not right" or "that sounds silly," but it's really important that you don't censor yourself.

The fact that some of the thoughts you write down don't seem to be in accord with reality, or the way you see things now, is actually part of the process. Later in this chapter, I'll discuss strategies for analyzing your negative automatic thoughts to determine whether they are realistic.

Making sure you've got all the thoughts you'll need. Before you move on to the next step, go back to the Thoughts column in your journal and try the following.

Read back the thoughts you recorded to yourself. Then, imagine that you are back in that situation again. If you feel the emotions you wrote down stirring up even a little bit, you've probably recorded the kinds of thoughts you actually had. Those emotions coming back to you, even in diminished form, tell you that those are the very same thoughts that connect your situation to the emotion. And that is the first, big, important step you can take when you are working with your thoughts, because a thought can be changed, and that change can help you to feel much better in the long run.

USING YOUR THOUGHT WORKSHEET TO MONITOR YOUR MOOD SHIFTS

The second step in the process of cognitive behavioral therapy is to look more closely at your thoughts in a specific situation. And you will expand the monitoring form that was introduced in the first step to help you do this. Remember that the kinds of thoughts that cause strong emotions, also known as *hot thoughts,* are often unrealistic, especially when you are already in a sad mood.

It's important to mention again that this doesn't mean the kinds of thoughts you are having are the cause of your depression. The ultimate cause of a depression can be a biological problem, most obviously an irregularity with your thyroid. Even so, if you are depressed, regardless of the cause, negative thoughts will be a part of your experience. If you can tackle those thoughts head-on and change them to be more in line with reality, you will be in a much better position to fight against your depression.

Using the Evidence to Discover the Truth

Evidence gathering is probably the most powerful method for discovering whether your thinking is realistic, and whether it fits the facts of the situation. Evidence gathering puts you in the position of becoming a more objective observer by having you carefully examine the *facts* of a situation. In addition, evidence gathering asks you to consider both the facts that may support your original interpretation (the hot thought) and those that support one or more alternative interpretations (alternative thoughts).

Ask yourself questions. Before you try some evidence gathering yourself, let's go back to the example of Kelly's nasty argument with her husband. Remember that in her situation, Kelly's husband had become upset when their daughter hurt herself, and Kelly had a thought that she found particularly distressing: "John thinks I'm a bad mother." Because she was involved in cognitive behavioral therapy, she realized that if she was going to try to gather evidence, she would have to step back a bit and ask some questions, including "What are the facts I know for sure?"

One fact she knew for sure was that John had gotten upset, and she remembered that he had questioned her about how carefully she was watching Katie. The next good question she asked herself was "Do the facts I know point to the idea that John believes I am a bad mother?"

Well, right away you can see that John didn't say that Kelly was a bad mother. It seems that because John asked whether Kelly was watching their daughter carefully, Kelly *inferred* he had implied she was a bad mother. Do you see the problem?

We all make leaps like this sometimes. Your boss wants to talk to you; right away you think you're in trouble for something. When others express frustration over something, we often take it as criticism of ourselves. It's always good to ask, "What might I be missing about this situation?" In this case, why else might John have said what he said?

It could be that John was upset and spoke as he did because of his own emotional response to Katie's physical pain. We all know that when we are upset we say things we do not mean. Also, it's possible that John felt guilty too, since he also could have been watching Katie more closely. So, there were other possible reasons for John having said what he said. Certainly, we know that getting Katie hurt caused John to become upset.

So, after thinking things through, Kelly ended up concluding that John's upset meant something quite different than she had thought at first. After considering the possible reasons that he had become upset, Kelly realized that it was because he loves Katie and watches out for her. That didn't let John completely off the hook: Kelly also concluded that John's accusation was out of bounds and not helpful.

Broaden your perspective. Another thing to consider when looking at evidence is to broaden your perspective on your automatic thoughts. In our example, let's say for the moment that John's question "were you watching her closely" really was aimed directly at Kelly's parenting abilities. So, in the CBT process, she would step back again and ask herself, "Even if he thinks that, does this mean it's true?"

In other words, even if you're the best parent who ever lived, is it always possible to prevent your child from hurting herself? The answer, as you probably know, is that when children play, sometimes they get hurt. Take it one step further; is there anything good about when a child gets hurt? Surely, no one wants to be unsympathetic about a child's pain, but these kinds of minor scrapes do serve the function of teaching children to be careful and learn what their limits are.

If we all didn't experience getting hurt sometimes, we'd all be in trouble because we would just continue doing more and more danger-ous things. So, a natural question to ask is this: "Would a good mother prevent her child from experiencing any pain at all?" The answer must be no, because no one can protect children so completely. Not allow-ing kids to play on slides, use playground equipment, or ride bikes will not teach kids about real life and real consequences. Note, too, this is not to say that you shouldn't take precautions; a helmet for bike riding is an excellent idea, but complete protection from any injury is not pos-sible and not, in fact, desirable.

Completing Your Thought Worksheet

So, now you are nearly ready to return to your journal to com-plete your thought worksheet. Open your journal to the blank page on the right-hand side and copy table 10.2: Sample Thought Worksheet (cont.). This page should be next to the page on which you copied the sample worksheet earlier in this chapter. This new table will have four columns with four headings: Evidence, Distortions, Alternative or Bal-anced Thought, and New Emotions. But before you start writing about your situation, please read the following sections that correspond to the headings in your new worksheet.

EVIDENCE

Generally, the idea with evidence is to step away from your usual, personal way of interpreting your thoughts and step back to try to become a more neutral, detached observer or judge. When using this

Table 10.2: Thought Worksheet (cont.)

Evidence	Distortions	Alternative or Balanced Thought	New Emotions

Table 10.2: Sample Thought Worksheet (cont.)

Evidence	Distortions	Alternative or Balanced Thought	New Emotions
John was upset and asked me whether I was watching her closely-in an angry tone.	Personalizing	John was upset and he shouldn't have spoken to me that way, but he did out of concern for our daughter.	Less sad and angry, feeling better about myself
That could have meant that he thought I was a bad mother.	Black and white thinking	It isn't possible or necessary to always prevent Katie from getting hurt.	
He may have been upset for Katie, maybe guilty.			
He spoke out of concern, not to undermine me.			
Even if he meant it, Katie's scrape was part of playing.			
Some hurts are part of learning and growing up, this says nothing about my mothering abilities.			

strategy, some people find it useful to imagine that they are putting their thought "on trial," and that they are the judge looking at both sides of a case.

The prosecutor's role involves identifying the facts that support the negative conclusion. The role of the defense involves examining the facts that do not support the hot thought, or that raise doubts about whether the hot thought is true. Sometimes, it is helpful to take the attitude of wanting to poke holes in the story of the prosecutor. That is, some facts that seem to support the hot thought may not be very rational or realistic. The judge can then weigh both sides of the story and come up with a fair verdict (usually the alternative thought).

When you start to gather evidence, here are some questions you should ask yourself:

- What are the facts?

- Are there some facts that support my hot thought?

- Are there some facts that don't support my hot thought?

- Are the facts supporting my hot thought ironclad or could they also support another thought?

- What's the big picture?

- What would I say to a loved one, or what questions would I encourage another person to ask?

In the evidence column, you will jot down your observations about the facts of your particular situation. So, here are some other ideas for questions that might be helpful to include in your evidence gathering:

1. **Get more information about the context.** What is the background of the situation? Are there reasons something is happening that aren't about me? Are there elements in this situation that I don't know or that are beyond my control or responsibility?

2. **Take a more objective view.** Would my best friend or a trusted family member see this the same way? What would I tell my best friend about this thought?

3. **Take a longer-range view of the situation.** How will I see this situation in a month, in a year, or five years from now?

Does the situation need to "develop" over time before I have a complete picture? Am I looking at just a single moment in time and not taking into account the longer term?

DISTORTIONS

It can be very useful to remember that *all* of our thoughts are occasionally subject to distortions or biases. Cognitive behavioral therapy involves helping people become attuned to these cognitive errors and tries to teach them how to catch such errors early in the process. This not only leads to more balanced thoughts (especially when coupled with evidence gathering), it also provides a quick way to become aware of your usual thinking patterns, and to learn what to look out for. Many people discover that they are prone to making the same kind of distortion across many different situations. If this is one of your mental habits, knowing that you are prone to making distortions can be really useful.

These errors in thinking, called *cognitive distortions*, occur when you don't take into account all of the information in a given situation. Some typical distortions include the following:

Arbitrary inference. This means coming to a specific conclusion without supporting evidence, or even in the face of contradictory evidence. *Example:* A harried worker trying to meet a deadline who cannot accomplish all of his or her tasks in one day thinking, "I'm a terribly inefficient employee."

Selective abstraction. This means seeing a situation in terms of a single detail taken out of context, and ignoring other information in the situation. *Example:* Focusing on a single piece of negative feedback from a performance evaluation that is otherwise filled with positive feedback, and then becoming sad and feeling hopeless.

Overgeneralizing. This means taking a rule that applies to one situation or perhaps to a few incidents, and applying it to situations in which the rule doesn't apply at all. *Example:* After having difficulty with a single unruly child in a class, a teacher concluded, "All of these children are rude, noisy, and ill-mannered."

Magnifying and minimizing. *Magnifying* involves seeing certain things (usually your own faults or flaws) as far more significant than they really are. *Example:* A woman on a first date unintentionally mentions that her former boyfriend left her, and then thinks to herself, "Now I've done it. Now he knows there's something wrong with me."

Minimizing involves seeing certain facts (usually someone else's flaws or faults) as far less significant than they really are. *Example:* Downplaying or ignoring the fact that your spouse has had an extra-marital affair, and perhaps even blaming yourself for what happened.

Personalizing. This means attributing external events to yourself, without any evidence to support such a causal connection. *Example:* At a party, a woman overhears someone saying that there aren't enough interesting people at the gathering, and she has the thought, "I know he's talking about me."

Dichotomous thinking or black-and-white thinking. This means categorizing experiences into one of two extremes (e.g., right or wrong, good or bad, complete success or total failure). *Example:* A woman who was cooking a family dinner believed that one of her side dishes had not turned out perfectly and thought, "The entire dinner is ruined."

Mind reading. This means to believe that you know what another person is thinking, despite a lack of any direct evidence. *Example:* While engaged in a conversation at a party, you assume that the other person finds the conversation boring, despite the fact that you have no evidence to support such an assumption.

Keeping this list of distortions in mind, let's return briefly to Kelly and John's situation. Kelly decided that she had been personalizing John's statements and his emotions as directed at her. When she really looked at the evidence, it seemed that much of what John said to her had been triggered because he was upset that their daughter had hurt herself and was in distress. Kelly also noted that she was thinking in black-and-white terms, e.g., that if she was a good mother, her child would never hurt herself, or that if she looked away from her daughter, even for even a few seconds, this meant that she was a bad mother.

When thinking about possible distortions you might have made in your analysis of the situation, asking yourself the following two questions can be very helpful:

- Is my thought a distortion?

- If so, what is the distortion?

Keeping these kinds of distortions in mind as you complete the thought worksheet in your journal will really help to change the direction your thoughts take you. With practice, the processes of evidence gathering and identifying distortions will become more efficient, especially after you've begun to identify some patterns in your thinking.

ALTERNATIVE OR BALANCED THOUGHT

Once you've arrived at a more complete picture of your situation and new thoughts emerge, you can write down a more balanced, alternative thought that takes into account the distortions and evidence that you've gathered. The chances are pretty good that these new thoughts and ways of looking at the situation will be much less emotionally upsetting than your hot thought was.

Remember, a hot thought is the kind of thought that causes strong emotions and is often unrealistic, especially when you are already in a sad mood. Some people struggle with trying to identify alternative, or more balanced thoughts. This struggle can be a sign that the automatic thought is more realistic than not. We'll deal with that in the next section.

In most circumstances, the simplest way to come up with an alternative or more balanced thought is to summarize all of the facts in the Evidence column, and then consider what distortion occurred. This will often suggest a new perspective on the entire experience.

Going back to Kelly and John's situation, Kelly had several new thoughts that gave her a different perspective on the experience: "John was upset and he shouldn't have spoken to me the way he did, but he did it out of his concern for our daughter," and "It isn't necessary or even possible to always prevent Katie from getting hurt."

When you are trying to come up with an alternative or more balanced thought about your particular situation, following the bulleted suggestions below can be very helpful:

■ Write down your new, alternative thought taking into account all of the evidence you've gathered and all of the distortions you may have made.

■ Your alternative thought should summarize everything you've discovered from the evidence and from any distortions.

NEW EMOTIONS

Once you've got a new balanced thought, or perhaps several new conclusions, ask yourself, "What are my feelings about the situation now?" Alternatively, look back at the original Emotions column and ask yourself, "With these new thoughts, would I still feel the same way?" If you're evidence gathering has gone well, and you've identified some distortions in your thoughts, you may feel quite differently. In some cases, not all the emotions will be completely gone, but most people writing a thought worksheet will see at least a 50 percent reduction in the intensity of their emotions. In Kelly's situation, her new emotions were "calm," and "accepting," but also "angry." We might understand that looking at evidence, it was clear that in no way was she a bad mother, and hence her hurt all but disappeared. But then why was she angry?

The anger reflected her frustration with her husband's response to the situation, his apparent accusation, and his tone. In fact, she planned to address the issue with him, so that he wouldn't speak to her in that way again, no matter how upset he was. This really is a sign of a successful thought worksheet. Not only did Kelly feel much better, but she also identified a communication problem that was actually solvable. The thought "I'm a bad mother" became a distant memory!

COMPLETING YOUR THOUGHT WORKSHEET

In practice, completing a thought worksheet can have two different outcomes.

You may uncover evidence that completely changes your hot thoughts. This can occur because asking yourself probing questions can reveal a whole new perspective or set of facts that directly contradict your hot thought. When you do find that your hot thought is definitely not true, it's often easy to come up with an alternative statement that reflects more of the truth in a given situation.

The second possible outcome is that the evidence gives you a "split decision." That is, when all the evidence is in, there's a chance your hot thought has some truth to it and, at the same time, you also have some evidence that there's more complexity to the situation, and your hot thought isn't the most logical conclusion.

In this second case, you may find that you need more information to test out whether your thought is true. In CBT, we call the process of seeking additional information to test out the truth of thoughts an *experiment*, and an experiment can be as simple as asking someone a question.

In Kelly and John's situation, it might have been useful for Kelly to ask John what he meant by his statements. If she suspected that he was implying that she was not a watchful, good mother, she might have asked him if that's what, in fact, he was trying to communicate.

The point of an experiment is to try to get more information that will tell you what is really going on. In Kelly and John's case, the experiment would have helped Kelly understand more about whether or not she was personalizing John's remarks excessively. And this is important, too: Kelly could also have used that opportunity to let John know that his statements had hurt her and were not very helpful to the situation.

Sometimes parts of our automatic or hot thoughts are true; after all, bad things happen to everyone from time to time. Losing a job can lead to financial struggles, the end of a relationship can involve a lot of heartache. In Kelly and John's case, let's assume that their marriage was already in trouble and John really was trying to undermine Kelly's sense of her self-worth, particularly in her role of mother. In that case, the situation and Kelly's own reaction should have been a signal to her that there was, indeed, a problem that needed to be addressed.

So, if or when you find yourself in a situation similar to Kelly and John's, and you've asked some hard questions to find out what is really going on, once you receive some answers, what is your next step?

The next step is to consider this question: "What can I do about it?" What are the active steps you can take to repair the situation or prevent it from continuing to happen? If this is a problem you have control over, you may also ask these questions:

■   What do the problem-solving steps look like?

■   When do I want to begin to problem solve?

■   What support do I need to solve the problem?

Chapter 11, concerned with stress, deals in-depth with larger stressors in ways that will also be useful to you when your automatic thoughts are partly true and point to a real problem.

Checking Your Mood

To complete your thought worksheet, your final step will be to check in with yourself again to see if you *feel* any differently about the situation once you've looked at it through this new lens of CBT practices. To do this, think again about how you felt at the time the situation occurred, focusing on the specific emotions you experienced. Now that you have more evidence, know whether there were distortions, and look again at your alternative thoughts, do you still feel the same way you did when you the situation originally occurred? Write down whatever changes you notice in the final column, New Emotions. This is the real payoff from these practices; most likely you will experience a positive change in your mood.

Summary

In this chapter, I've described the ideas behind CBT, which has proved to be very useful for coping with depression. In your depression, you've seen how your thinking can become biased and distorted, undermine your self-confidence, and lead to a range of negative emotions and problematic behaviors. I've also described how biological causes can spark changes in thinking and, just as importantly, how changing your thinking can change your biology.

This chapter has provided a step-by-step approach to help you observe your negative thoughts and moods. CBT has a simple but powerful kind of technology in the thought worksheet. Being able to use a thought worksheet on the fly in any situation that arises is probably one of the most helpful tools of the therapy. Combining the use of this kind of worksheet with other treatments, such as the correction of thyroid imbalances and the use of antidepressant medications, will be useful for recovering faster and more completely from depression.

Remember to practice these skills regularly. I fully expect readers will need to reread this chapter as they work on getting better by completing their thought worksheets. Remember, too, that if you have questions, a cognitive behavioral therapist who works in your area may be able to help you work out any kinks in your practice of these strategies.

CHAPTER 11

Stress

"Stress" is a very interesting word; in a way it's become a catchphrase of our times. We all think we know what stress is, and we seem to relate to having a lot of it in our lives. The media talks about stress frequently, usually attached to the idea that we need to return to a "simpler time," a time when there was less stress. This chapter is about stress too, because it's true that stress represents a real problem for many people, especially those who are vulnerable to depression and medical illnesses. But I want first to step back and take a more careful look at what stress is, to define the term a bit more precisely and to connect the dots between thyroid problems, depression, and stress.

WHAT IS STRESS?

I invite you to sit back just for a moment and contemplate this question: What is stress?3 What does the word mean to you? Perhaps the word brings up ideas about living life at too fast a pace; having too many obligations and not enough time; dealing with irritations and hassles every day; getting by in a world that cares about results, not people; living through a terrible event that turns us into survivors. Right away, you can see that the word "stress" covers a pretty broad area. It applies to everything from a car that won't start to dealing with a newly diagnosed terminal illness. The idea that stress is multiple things that happen for many reasons is useful, and it obviously leads to the idea that we need to have different responses to different kinds of stressors.

What do scientists and people who study stress mean when they use the term? Hans Selye (1978), considered by most scholars to be the father of stress studies, defined stress as any demand made on an animal that requires a physiological response. This more scientific version of stress is not only more precise than the definitions offered above, it also sheds light on the nature of stress in a way that goes beyond life's hassles and events. It adds the extremely important idea that when events happen, our bodies (and brains) have a set of built-in responses to deal with whatever that situation may require. The event causing stress can be trivial or profound. In Selye's theory, both an exercise workout and the death of a loved one can cause significant stress. What these events have in common is that they place a load or strain on the organism.

People who study the physiology of stress often work with animals so they can conduct careful experiments to study how the various systems in the body, such as hormones, neurons, and organs, respond to specific kinds of events. This important research, which we cannot do in humans, has helped us to understand more about how our biology is affected by stress.

So, if stress is nothing more than a strain on the body that requires a response, this can only mean that stress really is a normal part of living. Based on our evolutionary history, our bodies are carefully designed to respond to certain demands. For example, when an animal sees a predator, this will create a form of stress, but it is a "good" stress. The animal responds to the sight of a predator with a series of physiological responses that help it to defend itself or to run away. (This is often called the fight-or-flight response.)

If that was all there was to it, this would be fine. However, Selye, and others since his time, also observed that when there are too many stresses with which an animal must cope, the animal's physiological systems eventually will become overwhelmed, and lead to physical breakdowns. So, this additional fact leaves us with a bit of a balancing act. We cannot and should not try to avoid all stress. (Stress researchers say that even when we are sound asleep there may be certain loads or strains on the body.) Yet, too much stress, too many demands, strains, and loads can wear us down physically and mentally.

THE BRAIN, BODY, AND TOO MUCH STRESS

I've already made the point that the mind and body are very closely connected; nowhere is this more evident than when stress is discussed. The systems of the body that respond to fight-or-flight are classic examples of this deep connection.

Question: Let's suppose you are walking down a dark alley late at night, and you see a figure rushing toward you. What will your first response be? Answer: Your sympathetic nervous system will take over your body's functioning very quickly. Among other changes, your digestion will slow down and blood flow will be diverted from your digestive organs to the "action" muscles in your arms and legs; your heart rate will speed up to supply you with more energy; and much more brain activity will be focused on scanning for threats. Whatever you were thinking about before you saw the figure rushing toward you will likely vanish from your thoughts and you'll be ready to flee.

Now, that's an extreme example of a stress load but many other stresses we experience are just variations on similar physiological processes. This kind of stress, the sudden need to flee or fight, is undoubtedly less relevant to this book than "real life" stress. Nonetheless, it is useful to understand what stress does to body and brain because the physiological responses to stress are much the same, regardless of whether the stress is caused by a figure rushing toward you in a dark alley or fear of failing an important exam.

The short story about stress and the body is simple: ongoing stress has an enormous impact on hormones, brain development, and even brain structure and functioning. The long story about stress is, of course, fairly complex and involves a lot of detail about biological systems. There is such an inherent complexity in the brain-body connection that we end up with hundreds of studies, each researcher studying a small piece of the puzzle.

Stress hormones. For example, we know that stress hormones, which are released from a variety of glands located throughout the body, affect the brain. We also know that the hippocampus and the amygdala, two carefully studied parts of the brain, are important in processing stressors related to fear. But these parts of the brain also trigger certain glands to release the stress hormone cortisol (McEwen 1995). This means that when the mind has determined there is a stressor, the brain helps to trigger the release of hormones. We also know that these same stress hormones then bathe the brain, so there are some very complicated feedback loops going on.

Homeostasis. In fact, people who have physiological problems with hormone release do suffer emotional consequences, even in the absence of external stressors. One very useful way to think about stress is to think of it as a balance scale, with stress on one side and the body's response on the other. Our bodies try to balance the two naturally to arrive at a balance point (this point is called *homeostasis*, which means a relatively stable state of equilibrium).

So, if the body and brain always try to balance stress, why is stress bad for you? Well, think of a small weight (weighing 10 pounds perhaps) of stress and a small body-brain response, also weighing about 10 pounds to balance things out, and there is no problem. But then, consider a large weight of stress, say, the equivalent of 100 pounds; now the body must respond with the equivalent of 100 pounds of stress hormones. But now the entire metaphorical scale is burdened with a 200-pound load, whereas it was formerly a mere 20 pounds. Under which condition are you more likely to have a problem? Obviously, the heavier load will create more problems because now the balance is harder to achieve. The whole scale could collapse and any imbalance will create a very unstable situation.

Allostatic load. Researchers call this general idea about balance the *allostatic load* (McEwen 1995). Too much allostatic load can defeat what is sometimes called the "wisdom of the body." It's true that, most of the time, our bodies respond to stress in ways that help us to handle stressful events; these ways activate us to fight back, and they prepare us to deal with threats. But when too much stress is experienced for too long, the body's response starts to work against itself.

For example, by a complex series of events hardwired into our biology, human beings undergoing a great deal of stress end up signaling their bodies to retain more fat, thus making our bodies unhealthier, more vulnerable to heart disease, and, probably in the long run, less efficient at dealing with stress. Depression in particular seems to increase *cortisol* levels (cortisol is a stress hormone related to adrenaline), and wears down the body's resistance to a host of illnesses (McEwen 1995).

Some of the hormones involved in the stress response actually suppress the immune system, thus making us more vulnerable to autoimmune problems and to fever (McEwen 2003). These same hormones also contribute to muscular atrophy and to calcium loss from our bones (McEwen 2003). So, although it's true that the body is capable of reacting to and dealing with stressors on most occasions, a too heavy allostatic load is the hidden price we pay much of the time (McEwen 1995).

There is also compelling evidence that stress is associated with triggering hyperthyroidism, also called Graves' disease (Winsa et al. 1991), and that stress can undermine the treatment of thyroid problems with medications (Fukao et al. 2003). So, we know that the thyroid gland does indeed respond to stress and can, in fact, be overwhelmed by stress. Furthermore, we know that medical treatment alone may not be sufficient to reverse the problem. Therefore, for the health of the thyroid gland, and the health of our bodies, in general, we need to look at how we deal with stress in order to reduce it more effectively.

STRESS AND DEPRESSION

Independent of the research on biological factors associated with stress, we've known for more than twenty years that stress is strongly tied to depression (Billings, Cronkite, and Moos 1983). People who are clinically depressed, typically, will have as many as three times the number of stressors in their lives than people who are not depressed.

There are both psychological and biological reasons why stress results in depression; and, in fact, both mental and physical mechanisms do come into play. In a sense, the erosion of someone's psychological capacities has some of the same effects as the erosion of that person's physical capacities; certainly, one interacts with the other in both the brain and the body.

What Is a Stressor?

Getting down to the more practical aspects of this discussion, typically, stress is associated with certain kinds of life events. What are the kinds of events that cause us to respond with the highest stress levels? It turns out that even this simple question contains some subtle paradoxes. There are disagreements in the psychological literature about what kind of event ought to be defined as a stressor (Monroe and Simons 1991).

EXTERNAL EVENTS AND DAILY HASSLES

Some people think we should call something a stressor only if there is a clearly defined external event (e.g., a medical illness, the death of a loved one, the loss of a job, a divorce or separation, becoming a victim of a crime). People on this side of the argument say that if we confine ourselves to these "big" events, we can better study the relationship between negative life events and depression (Monroe and Simons 1991).

There are, however, other researchers who think we also need to study smaller events, sometimes called *daily hassles.* These researchers believe that the way in which the person perceives a situation is what makes it a stressor. In this view, someone trapped in a massive traffic jam who manages to stay cheerful by listening to her favorite music doesn't perceive the traffic jam as a stressor; whereas someone late for a meeting with her boss, who is caught in the same traffic jam, would perceive it as a major stressor. In this view almost anything could count as a stressor; in other words, stress is in the eye of the beholder. If there is a problem with this definition, it's that almost any situation can be defined a stressor, even minor irritations like being unable to find your house keys or having to wait in a long line to get into a movie theater.

But for us to progress in our understanding of stress we need to use both definitions. That's because both sides have excellent arguments. Clearly, there are some events that will always cause some degree of stress; for example, getting a divorce has been shown to be one of the biggest life stressors related to psychological distress. No one getting a divorce is immune from some level of stress. However, the amount and type of stress might differ.

For example, if the reason someone seeks a divorce is that he no longer loves his wife, and has fallen in love with someone else, he will have a very different experience of divorce when compared to his wife, who is "being left." He might feel some guilt and shame, but he will also feel some relief and will eagerly anticipate his future. The person being left is more likely to be hurt, angry, possibly self-critical, and feel a strong sense of abandonment.

Which person has more stress? Even in a situation like this, where it might seem easy to say who experiences the most stress, just based on the facts, it is actually difficult to answer. That's because so much also has to do with the personalities of the people. So, stress is both an external event and something that affects each person in a unique manner.

REPETITIVE STRESSES

Also important is the fact that the most common stressors based on how frequently they occur are, in fact, not the big events that strike out of the blue. Instead, the most common stressors are the ones that are part of daily life; events that if they took place just once in a while, would probably not be a big deal, but because they are repetitive and because that repetition is beyond our control, they wear down the body and mind in significant ways. We've called these kinds of stressors daily hassles, and they too cause strain.

Consider how a landscape changes over time. Certainly, earthquakes (out-of-the-blue, big stresses) reshape the land; but over time a simple stream of water that doesn't look especially powerful will carve a deep, significant valley. So, having to drive every day in rush-hour traffic, work every day at a high-pressure job, and deal every day with ongoing conflicts with people we love are also significant life events that place a heavy load of stress on our minds and bodies.

Two different sets of issues. We then have two very different types of issues to deal with. The first is what to do when something unfortunate befalls us. For example, we lose a job, get separated, or suffer the loss of a loved one. These are stressors we must cope with and find ways to come to terms with. The second issue is the daily hassles we endure, because these too are areas we can influence. Sometimes, we can find ways around the difficulties, and sometimes we can find ways to be more at peace with them, even when these are distasteful things we wish we didn't have to experience.

Keep in mind that many events and ways to deal with them fall right in the middle; that is, they are neither big, out-of-the blue events, nor daily hassles. There is no one universally "right" strategy for dealing with stressors. For example, if someone you love were to be diagnosed with a serious illness, that would be a big stressor; but let's also say that over time that person will not be in mortal danger, but will require difficult treatment and rehabilitation. In such a case, the initial shock of stress would turn into a more chronic situation; one that you would have to continue dealing with on a daily basis. In fact, the reality is that you will want to try to mix and match various strategies for the stressors you experience. And, remember, your thyroid gland (and all your hormonal systems) will thank you.

DEALING WITH BIG STRESSORS

Usually, big stressors are those that come as a shock; indeed, their surprise element may be why we react so strongly to them. What kinds of events count as "big"? Well, questionnaires designed to assess stress can help with this. I've listed eleven possible big stressors below. Taken from a combination of stress inventories, they are as follows:

1. Death of a child, spouse, parent, close friend, or relative

2. Diagnosis of a serious medical illness and disability

3. A family member diagnosed with a serious medical illness

4. Becoming a caregiver for a sick person

5. Separation/Divorce

6. Getting married

7. Having a child

8. Losing a job and being unemployed

9. Serious financial losses

10. Moving or having a family member move away

11. Retirement

Obviously, each of these events would be uniquely distressing if they happened to any of us tomorrow. And all of them would create instant stress. There is no doubt that having strong emotional and physical reactions to events like these is entirely normal. Such a response (think back to the earlier definition of stress attributed to Hans Selye) is completely in line with humanity's evolutionary past, and is simply the body getting ready with a response.

Does this mean there's nothing you can do? In one sense, it's true that it's important to allow yourself to feel the feelings you are having. For example, at the end of a romantic relationship, some people will tell themselves that they ought not to feel sad or ought not cry. In this case, it might be more common for a man to think, "I shouldn't cry," and thus suppress his emotions about a breakup or divorce. So, it is definitely important to not get in the way of a normal stress reaction and just let it happen.

On the other hand, stress reactions sometimes last longer than is ideal, and the choices people make about what they do about a stressor can be important. Depending on the "size" of the stressor, most people feel better after a few months, or sometimes a little longer. If you feel as though things haven't improved much one year after a big stressor has occurred in your life, you should probably seek professional advice.

COPING STRATEGIES

Most often, the ways we respond to stressors are called *coping*. This is an entirely different research area that branches off from the study of stress. The number of things that people do to deal with stress is probably infinite; they range from eating comfort food, to crying, to writing in a diary, to working out at the gym. Anything can be considered a coping strategy if the stressed-out person sees the activity he or she is engaged in as helping to defuse or get through stress.

Active and passive strategies. The question to ask is this: What kinds of coping strategies work and what kinds don't? We have some pretty good answers to these questions but, even then, some things might work for one person and not for another. One of the most helpful ways to think about coping strategies is whether they are active or passive. *Active* describes actions you might take to tackle a problem; *passive* refers to strategies that have more to do with experiencing the stress, like talking about the problem with other people, thinking about how it makes you feel, and expressing your emotions about it. It's true that people under stress need to experience and talk about their problems, freely expressing their emotions. But we also know that overreliance on the more passive strategies tends in the long run not to be helpful (Cronkite and Moos 1995).

Escaping and ruminating. Many depressed people tend to use too much "escape" coping (i.e., trying to distract themselves too much or pretending that the problem doesn't exist). Escaping is a form of emotional avoidance. It may involve talking around the problem rather that getting to the heart of it. Talking about a problem can also end up triggering rumination, a well-known risk factor for depression (Nolen-Hoeksema 2000). *Rumination* is best described as thinking or worrying about an event in a manner that goes around in circles—spinning your wheels—without ever getting to any kind of forward motion.

People who ruminate get lost in their thoughts, perhaps magnifying particular parts of a problem and not seeing the potential for ways out of whatever dilemma they are in (see chapter 10 for cognitive strategies). Also, no amount of discussion or thought can help to solve a problem in the absence of actual behavior aimed at solving the problem. Sometimes, tackling a problem that results from a stressor is the absolute priority.

Coping with Divorce

Let's look at a specific example to take this discussion from theory into practice. One of the items on the list of big stressors above is separating or getting a divorce. Divorce is not an uncommon stressor; it's not an everyday issue, of course, but it's a significant possibility for anyone who is married or living with a domestic partner. Why is divorce so stressful in the first place?

The complete answer probably involves both evolution and culture. As with many animals, having a mate is perhaps the most critical priority for human beings; it is how we procreate. Some mammals, including humans, have a clear propensity to choose long-term mates (though not always lifelong). Moreover, our culture reflects this; we honor the institution of marriage as an "ideal state"; falling (and staying) in love is a cultural touchstone in popular culture as well as in all the arts.

Think about it. In the movies, single people are always on their way to that better state of being in love. We instinctively feel sorry for people who are alone. Matchmaking and falling in love are perhaps the most consistent themes in Western literature. Even when marriages fail, most people remarry despite the pain of having lived through a divorce. So, being married—or at least pair-bonded—seems to represent an ideal state for human beings, and the sudden absence of your mate, whether it is up to you or not, will be perceived in your mind and body as a stressor and, therefore, will result in a stress load on your mind and body.

The pain of a divorce is unavoidable. No matter how friendly or amiable the divorce agreement is, in its wake there will be sadness, anger, and loneliness; stress hormones will be released; we will feel different than our usual selves and we will also act differently than we would under most other circumstances. For some, divorce can trigger an episode of clinical depression; they may consider using antidepressants or seek counseling. But what is the best way to cope with the stressor of divorce?

THREE GOOD WAYS TO COPE

There are three categories of coping that are relevant here: emotion-focused coping, distraction coping, and problem solving. Although these three strategies are especially useful when dealing with a divorce, they are also very helpful in other stressful situations. These three are all discussed in much greater detail later in this chapter. They are introduced here, however, because their relevance to this section is essential.

1. **Distraction coping** is an active form of coping. The goal of distraction is to take your mind away from a stressor and focus it on something else. This can range from tiny to grand events; i.e., from going out to see a movie to taking a vacation in a foreign land. Distraction provides a kind of mental break.

2. **Problem solving** is exactly what it sounds like. Many stressors provide us with thorny dilemmas that must be resolved, obstacles that prevent us from living the lives we want to live. Usually, problem solving is active and hands-on; it often makes us focus on the practical things that need to be accomplished.

3. **Emotion-focused coping** means contemplating how you feel about something, seeking a better understanding of why you feel the way you do, and sharing those emotions in discussions with others.

For most big stressors, including divorce, one single approach to stress reduction will probably not do the job. What is needed instead is a thoughtful balance combining these three approaches. Overreliance on only one approach can lead to a deepening of the stress reaction, possibly prolonging and, in some cases, adding to a strong negative emotional reaction.

For example, if you are getting divorced, it won't be particularly useful to rely exclusively on distraction coping. In fact, it's probably pretty clear that you can't cope with a divorce by going to see a lot of movies, or even by taking a vacation in Paris. But what if you relied entirely on emotion-focused coping? That, too, might not be ideal. Yes, you would understand your emotions and needs better, but divorce also brings about a whole series of practical problems: Where will you live? What are the legalities of your situation? How will your rights be protected? Questions like these are highly practical and they need to be dealt with by problem solving; no amount of emotion-focused coping will keep you fed, clothed, and with a roof over your head.

Not dealing adequately with practical matters has its own risks. Failing to deal with your practical legal and financial matters could also prolong your difficulties and even cause them to worsen. For example, people who don't deal competently with the legal aspects of their divorce could easily wind up in a one-down position compared to their former partners. This, in turn, can affect their ability to put their lives back together and move forward.

A BALANCED APPROACH

Too often when people are struggling to cope with a big stressor, it's because they are working with an incorrect balance of their coping strategies. Indeed, big stressors require a judicious combination of *all three* types of strategies. All individuals who go through the process of getting divorced will have strong emotional reactions and will have to consider carefully how they feel about their situation and what their needs are. Perhaps they will also need therapeutic support and counseling to cope with their strong emotions.

Those people who don't want to deal with their strong feelings through emotion-focused coping may be suppressing their emotions. And the chances are good that this kind of suppression can actually prolong the length of time they will need to really recover from the stress of getting divorced. But they will also need to do some fairly intensive problem solving; perhaps most of their time will have to be spent dealing with the practicalities of creating new lives for themselves.

Finally, some amount of distraction coping will be called for; there will be times when the best thing you can do for yourself will be to give yourself a break and have some kind of fun. Having fun, even when the pressure is intense, will give you a mental break. These breaks can be crucial because often they sharpen our other abilities. Working with big stressors is real work, and just as with real work, we are all at our best when we take breaks and return to our work refreshed and with a positive outlook.

So, all this is meant to emphasize this simple but powerful point: Coping with stressors requires a careful balance of coping strategies, and if matters aren't going as well as you had hoped, consider changing the balance of the coping strategies you are using. In a divorce situation, the exact balance will differ depending on your unique needs and some of the situation-specific factors. This fact prevents me from recommending an ideal mix of strategies for everyone.

Nevertheless, if you are dealing with a big stressor, a good rule of thumb would be to spend about 45 percent of your time on problem solving, 45 percent on emotion-focused discussion, and 10 percent on distracting activities. Try to remember that whenever a stressor starts to overwhelm you, it is most likely time to examine the relative balance of the coping strategies you are using. That is far more important than adhering to any arbitrary division of coping strategies.

1. DISTRACTION COPING

Essentially, this type of coping involves occupying your mind with something other than your problem; that is, engaging in stimulating things to change your emotional state and the focus of your attention. In this category, you can include just about any activity that draws your attention away from your problem. Often, these are actions that are in and of themselves engaging and tend to activate positive emotions. For example, movies are engaging because they draw us out of ourselves into the world of the characters and story. But physical activity can also be distracting and helpful; for example, most sports require us to concentrate on the activity and, in a sense, to change our mental priorities while we are engaged with them. Here are some examples of distraction-avoidance coping in response to a stressor:

- Going to a movie or play; watching TV

- Sports, individual and team (Watching sports is good but playing them is even better.)

- Sleeping or napping

■ Pampering your body, i.e., treating yourself to a spa treatment or massage

■ Going to a party or club to dance and have fun

■ Leaving town to visit a new place

■ Hanging out with friends or loved ones

■ Using a computer to explore the world of cyberspace

■ Cleaning, or other household chores

As stated above, distraction coping strategies usually have nothing to do with the stressor. That is really where their power comes from because distractions should help you to unload your mind for a time. In fact, these strategies tend to work best if they are on the opposite side of the stressor's range. For example, if you are very stressed about your divorce, it may not be very distracting to go to a nightclub. That kind of milieu might trigger thoughts about relationships, especially yours, and it would not provide time off from your stressor at all.

What you want from a distraction is for your mind to be focused on the distracting activity you are engaged with right then, not focused on the stressor. It's important to remember that distractions can be light and fun, and that time off during a stressful period will always be necessary. Remember, too, that distractions can be a very important way of taking care of yourself so that you can recharge your energies to deal with whatever life brings to you.

The downside to these strategies is that they don't help you to come to grips with your stressor, make progress in understanding your feelings, or solve any problems. But this is the case with all coping strategies; each has a strength and a weakness, and each must be used in certain proportions and at certain times.

2.   PROBLEM SOLVING: TAKING ACTION

In this more action-oriented way of dealing with stressors, you reduce your stress by resolving the issues that result from the stressor. Often, this goes directly to the source of the problem and can involve gathering more information, as well as all manner of behaviors aimed at fixing or lessening the impact of the stressor. Taking an action-oriented way might include doing things like the following:

- Trying to find out more about the situation, especially what you can do to help yourself

- Getting professional advice or searching for information that will be a guide to decision making

- Talking to others who have had the same or a similar problem to see what they did about it

- Making a list of things that could be done about the problem

- Taking steps to resolve the problem

- Working on finding the most logical solution to the problem

Problem-solving strategies are at the heart of most of our action coping behaviors. Action-oriented coping tends to involve less emotion and more logic, more effort and less reflection. These strategies are useful for fixing problems and finding solutions. In the earlier example of getting divorced, it was obvious that someone in that situation will have to deal with a complex set of emotional reactions. But all of the practical aspects of a divorce must also be resolved, in a sense, without reference to how you might feel. You'd need a place to live, a lawyer to protect your rights and entitlements, a plan to see your children. It almost doesn't matter how you feel about it; if you don't take care of these basic needs, the situation could become much, much worse.

The limitations of taking action are that problem solving alone doesn't take your feelings into account. If you take action without properly understanding your emotional life, you are likely to make significant mistakes. So, in a divorce situation, everyone is likely to need someone to represent their rights (a lawyer), but how will you instruct that lawyer? What is important to you right now? What would make you feel less distressed about the divorce?

In short, what are your needs? Problem solving, by itself, cannot answer these deeper questions. To know exactly what to do, you also need to understand yourself and your emotions in a meaningful way. That is where emotion-focused strategies come in.

3.   EMOTION-FOCUSED COPING

Emotion-focused coping also defines a broad range of experiences that help us to better understand ourselves and come to grips with our needs and desires. This kind of coping helps us to express our feelings, and by so doing, often deepens our insight into ourselves. Examples of emotion-focused coping follow:

- Sharing the way the problem makes you feel with someone you trust

- Exploring your feelings about the problem

- Getting support from other people

- Attending counseling or a therapeutic facility

- Allowing yourself to express your emotions, including crying

- Engaging in meditative practices

All of these behaviors have the potential to help you understand your feelings and the reasons why you are having such feelings. And they point the way to what you'll need to start doing to feel better. In fact, without emotion-focused coping, your other coping strategies may be less effective than they should be—all logic but lacking the emotional wisdom required for them to be really effective. Also, emotion-focused coping may involve other people offering their support. This is useful not only because they may offer good advice, but also because they may bring a new perspective to your problem. Other people may provide a whole new way of looking at the issue that could prove to be very helpful.

The downside to emotion-focused coping is that doing too much of this can become overwhelming or, even worse, can send you into a negative emotional spiral. Some people get very caught up in their feelings, and they can become overly focused on what is the "right" thing that must be done. Dealing with that kind of uncertainty, however, can cause you to become stuck, especially if you are not doing at least a few practical problem-solving actions.

In a worst case scenario, if you use only emotion-focused coping to deal with a large stressor, you risk extending your suffering needlessly. Emotions can be ethereal, hard to pin down, and by their very nature difficult to define with any degree of certainty. Therefore, it makes sense to combine action-oriented coping with emotionally focused coping, using your emotions as a guide or compass, and the action as your forward motion toward your goals. Corrections to the course will be needed, via waypoints that will help you check and correct your course when necessary.

MAKING A COPING PLAN THAT WORKS FOR YOU

Now, to learn how to use coping strategies in different problem situations, pick up your journal and open it to two blank facing pages. You will be using a step-by-step approach. Note that large problems (like a financial crisis) are likely to require you to use the three types of coping strategies in different "doses."

Be sure to leave yourself plenty of space to write in. This exercise may spill over to four, six, or even eight pages. That's fine. The more details you write, the more benefits will result from doing the exercise.

EXERCISE 11.1: THE COPING WORKSHEET

1. My **goal** or the **problem** I am trying to cope with is:

   _____

   The consequences of this goal or problem are:

   _____

2. **Emotion-focused coping.** Ask yourself these questions: "To what extent can emotion-focused coping help me with the consequences I listed in step 1? What kind of emotion-focused strategies can I use?" Then, answer these questions using as many examples of emotion-focused strategies as you can come up with.

3. **Distraction coping.** Ask yourself this question: "To what extent can distraction coping help me with the consequences I listed in step 1?" Then, answer this by listing as many distraction coping strategies that you can imagine.

4. **Action-oriented coping.** Ask yourself: "To what extent can action-oriented coping help me with the consequences I listed in step 1?" Then, answer this question with as many possibilities for actions that you can imagine as realistic.

5. **Balancing your strategies.** This is the final step. Based on your previous answers, what proportion of your coping strategies should be given to each type of strategy? Again, ask

yourself how distraction, emotion-focused, and action-oriented strategies can help you with the consequences you listed in step 1. Then, when you've assigned percentages, say, 15 percent to distractions, 30 percent to emotion-focused strategies, and 55 percent to action-oriented strategies, you will have a plan that will help you to solve the problem you listed in step 1.

You can use this step-by-step process for any number of problems or goals you may have. The more often you work out the answers to these kinds of questions, the easier and more useful the whole process will become for you.

Remember, emotion-focused coping is used to clarify your feelings; if necessary, you can take the time to grieve a little, but also to establish what you want to do in the future. Action-oriented coping is used to pursue practical problem-solving options, and distraction is used to make sure you are not preoccupied twenty-four hours a day with your goal or problem.

Note: Each of the coping behaviors is supposed to have a different goal. If you are thinking of using a coping behavior, but you can't specify what the goal of that behavior is, you might be better off selecting another behavior or a different strategy altogether.

Record the strategy's limits. It is also wise to record what the limits of the three types of coping strategies might be for a particular situation. For example, neither emotion-focused coping nor distraction coping will help you find a new job. Moreover, even though action-oriented coping used by itself might help you to find a job, it would not necessarily be a job with an ideal fit, given your individual abilities and specific desires. Your emotion-focused and distraction coping strategies could be helpful in refining your job search to find employment that would not only pay your bills but also provide you with some creative satisfactions and pleasures.

Balance your strategies. Remember, the bottom line is that effective coping is composed of a variety of strategies that must be balanced to be maximally effective. The next section focuses specifically on the issue of problem solving, which is perhaps the largest component of action-oriented coping, and one that often pays the biggest dividends.

PROBLEM-SOLVING STRATEGIES

Throughout this discussion of coping, the notion of problem solving has repeatedly come up. Today, we know that problem solving is linked to depression; in fact, some theorists have described deficiencies in the ability to solve problems as a core aspect of depression (Nezu 1987). In stressful situations, our hardwired hormonal and physical reactions often get in the way of effective problem solving. Many scientists now believe that our fight-or-flight reactions to threats often place us at a distinct disadvantage in the modern world.

Let's take a simple example. Suppose you've been called into your boss's office to discuss an issue about your work performance; specifically, your boss has some negative feedback to give you regarding a project you recently supervised.

Even reading such a scenario and imagining the scene has probably already triggered subtle changes in your brain functioning. In real life, such changes would be even more pronounced; the chances are your heart would race faster than usual, you might feel hot and flushed, your palms might be sweaty. This would be the classic stress reaction, nature's way of preparing you either to run away or, literally, leap at your boss to counterattack. Blood would be flowing to your big muscle groups, your digestion would stop, your senses would become keener and sharper. And yet, at the same time, you would recognize how useless most of these reactions are in this twenty-first century context. Neither fleeing nor fighting would be useful options for you in this situation.

Instead, what you would need would be to activate the parts of your brain that govern logical thought. Your challenge would be an intellectual one. How could you respond to your boss's negative feedback in a way that would represent your leadership of the project in the best possible light? If she is critical about your performance, how can you let her know that you accept her criticism, that you had intended differently, and that you believe you can improve next time? In any case, it would be your thinking brain, not your biceps, that would get you out of this situation unscathed.

So, in the case of psychological stress, we have to take into consideration the fact that nature and evolution might not be as helpful to us as we might wish. In fact, the response that would be the most helpful is the direct opposite of what our bodies would be preparing for, that is, to take a deliberate stance of calmness to assess the situation, fully understand what it means, and then take what we call "skillful" action. So, in the next section I'll describe a sequence to follow to keep yourself on track, in order to arrive at the best possible course of action.

What Is the Problem: What Do You Need?

Before you can take any action to help yourself, you need to know what you want from the situation. Where would you like to go with the situation. What would make it turn out in the best possible way? The trouble is that stressful situations tend to put us into overly emotional states that make it difficult to see things clearly, undermining our ability to make good decisions for ourselves.

Emotional numbing. Some people respond to stress with emotional numbing. They become stressed-out by being only vaguely aware of their distress. But suppressing your emotions also can be dysfunctional. Certainly, being out of touch with your emotions can prevent you from understanding yourself and your needs. So, before working with the mechanics of problem solving it's important to take stock; to figure out where you are now and where you need to go.

Where do you want to go? Sometimes, it can be useful to seek the help of a professional or, at least, the assistance of someone whose wisdom and input you trust, to clarify your needs. Other times, it is simply a matter of spending some time getting in touch with yourself and your specific needs. For this, some quiet contemplation, perhaps meditation, might be indicated.

Meditation. A complete discussion of the benefits of meditation is beyond the scope of this book, but meditation doesn't have to involve any kind of religious conversion or trips to Asia. In fact, scientists are increasingly interested in meditation as a practice that can alter brain and mental states; for example, mindfulness meditation appears to be effective in preventing relapse of depression (Segal, Williams, and Teasdale 2002). For detailed information on mindfulness practices and their benefits, there are a number of excellent books you can find easily. In my opinion, the best is Jon Kabat-Zinn's *Full Catastrophe Living* (1990). To acquaint you with the usefulness of mindfulness practices, here is an overview of how they might help you to deal with stress.

MINDFULNESS

What does *mindfulness* mean? Put simply, to be mindful is to pay attention to your experiences in a specific way. The idea is to simply "be with" the present moment of your experiences, whatever they might be. This sounds easy, but actually it's not easy at all. Our minds tend, by their very nature, to run off on tangents in a number of directions; they tell us stories about yesterday and tomorrow; they judge our experiences as "good" or "bad"; and they operate on a kind of automatic pilot. Under stress, this can keep us in a mental state that emphasizes worrying and ruminating, rather than serenity and insight. So, to help yourself begin to problem solve, you might try adopting some of the important attitudes of mindfulness.

Four attitudes are essential parts of being more mindful, and all four are excellent to adopt, especially when you are under stress. One easy way to start practicing and adopting these attitudes is to sit quietly in a stable posture for a short period of time, say ten minutes, and pay attention to the way your thoughts come and go. You needn't assume a difficult posture. Just be sure your feet are flat on the ground and that you are comfortable. You don't have to count your breaths, or close your eyes, although both of these practices can help you to stay seated and aware. What you want to do is sit quietly and watch your thoughts as they come and go.

Nonjudging. The first attitude is nonjudging, described by Kabat-Zinn (1990) as being an impartial witness to your own experience. If you watch your mind, that is, if you watch your thoughts come and go, for a time, you are likely to find that your mind is full of judgments about your experiences, usually along the dimensions of good and bad. You then tend to welcome "good" thoughts and feelings and you try to banish "bad" or aversive thoughts and feelings. Try not to get stuck on judging them as either good or bad. To really get in touch with yourself means that it is best simply to let whatever is happening "be."

Patience (nonstriving). The second attitude to work toward in mindfulness practice is patience, which is a kind of nonstriving. You just sit patiently and watch your thoughts go by without getting involved in them. Many people just starting to learn to be more mindful become frustrated with how difficult practicing this kind of patience can be; experienced meditators know that their minds will take off in one direction or another often. Remember, there is no particular place you are trying to get to. Just pay attention to your thoughts as they arise. Don't get caught up in them.

One common misperception that people new to this practice often have is that they want to achieve an advanced state of relaxation or "bliss." Indeed, this can be part of the experience; but at the beginning, there is mostly the physical discomfort of sitting still without moving, or the difficult emotions that come up for you that you try to stay with, without judging.

Acceptance. The third attitude to cultivate in mindfulness is acceptance. Whatever happens during an exercise is what happens during that exercise. Whatever thoughts or feelings arise in your moment-to-moment experience is what happens; no more and no less.

Letting go. The final attitude, related to the other three, is letting go. Letting go is all about not trying too hard to go anywhere or being determined to have something "special" happen.

Mindfulness meditation puts these attitudes to use in specific exercises that involve the breath, body, and movement. If you are interested in these practices, we urge you to read more about them in Jon Kabat-Zinn's work. But for the purposes of this chapter, cultivating these four attitudes in yourself and allowing time for mindfulness practice when your life is stressful will be important. Being mindful will give you another place from which to observe your experiences. It can put you in touch with yourself and your needs in a unique way.

SKILLFUL MEANS

When you choose to take action after a period of mindfulness, often you will end up using what are sometimes called "skillful means." These are ways to deal with problems that are informed and influenced by your wiser, often more focused and calm mind. So, once you know that you've contemplated what it is you want, it's time to turn to the practical aspects of problem solving, which always start with writing down what it is you need or want; in other words, what your goal is. This is the first formal step of problem solving (Mueser 1998).

Once you know where you need to get to, or what it is you need to cope with, your second step is to generate solutions, or ways to try to get to that outcome. The third step is to pick the best of the possible solutions by carefully weighing the pros and cons, and by figuring out which way of dealing with your problem is the most realistic and will have the greatest chance for success. Finally, you will need a fourth step in which you examine how well your solutions are turning out. Many times, when we get into problem solving, we need to tweak and update our methods on a continual basis. We will consider each one of these steps in turn and provide some specific instructions on how to go about doing them.

Defining Your Terms

It can help a lot to define your goals carefully to figure out what it is you need. For example, if you are in a stressful relationship and things aren't going well, and you'd like to work on improving them, it's important to know specifically what it is you want from your relationship. Do you want to increase your level of intimacy? And, if so, do you mean physical or emotional intimacy, or both? So, you'll need to ask yourself these questions:

- How do I want things to be?

- Who is part of the problem and who is part of the solution?

- What can I control, and how do I want to control it?

At this point, it would be a good idea to write your goal down so that you have a record of it, and can look at it again later to modify it, or track your progress. So, take out your journal and turn to two blank facing pages and get ready to do the next exercise.

EXERCISE 11.2: SOLUTION PLANNING

Like the previous exercise, this is done in a step-by-step manner. The first thing to write is, of course, what the specific stress is that you need to deal with. As before, give yourself plenty of room. It doesn't matter how many pages it takes. What does matter is to be as thorough and complete as you know how to be.

DEFINING THE PROBLEM

1. The first step is to describe the stressor that you are working with. It can be helpful to keep this description short and simple.

2. Then, ask yourself the following questions to specify your ultimate goal:

    ■   How do I want things to be in the future with respect to this problem?

    ■   What is a realistic goal for me with respect to this problem?

    ■   What do I need to arrive at a better place?

BRAINSTORMING SOLUTIONS

Now that you know what your problem is and you have a better sense of where you need to go, it's time to free up your mind to generate ideas. This is where meditation can be so helpful, because the first rule of brainstorming is that there are no rules, and when you practice mindfulness, your mind can come up with all manner of new ideas.

When we are stressed and confronted by problems, we often get trapped in our thoughts, we ruminate, we worry, we go around and around in mental circles and can't find our way out. But if we focus on what we want, quiet our minds, and are encouraged to think creatively, often we see new options. This is sometimes called "divergent thinking" because it actually does help us to do a sort of end run around our usual thoughts.

So, the trick (it really isn't a trick) is to just let your mind roam and come up with any idea at all. In fact, the more "out there" the idea is, the better. In other words, any idea is fair game and no solution should be judged as good or bad. Doing this part should seem more like an art than a science. Be sure to give yourself the time and space to really get into this, and generate as many ideas as you can. Remember that a wildly imaginative and completely impractical idea, after you write it down, might trigger a more realistic and doable idea that will be a good one. You may even find that this process can be fun and inspiring, but you must let go of your usual assumptions to get there.

PICKING THE RIGHT SOLUTION

When you have a nice long list of options and see that there are many possibilities, you may even feel a little better about your problem. At that point, it's time to switch your creative hat for a more rational, objective chapeau. First start by rearranging the ideas you gathered from brainstorming into a smaller set of categories. Then ask yourself these critical questions:

- How practical is each of these options?

- Could that option actually be followed?

- What do I need to make that option work?

- Does that option, in reality, have a fatal flaw?

- What are the consequences of carrying out that option, both good and bad?

What needs to be established is how practical a solution is and how many advantages and drawbacks it has. Worthwhile options must be practical, have some advantages, and few disadvantages. Whatever option best fits those criteria then moves to the top of your list.

IT'S ALL ABOUT THE FOLLOW-THROUGH

After you finish brainstorming, you will have a list of alternatives, and even some sense of which set of options will be the most likely to succeed. These are the guidelines for success that you'll need, but the next step is even more important: implementing your ideas. For most of us, this is the hardest part. Many of the world's problems have been solved on paper, but a paper solution is never enough for real change. We need to commit ourselves to action because that's how problems move from being troubling to being resolved. Also, once we start to follow a solution, we learn relatively quickly what will work and where we need to make adjustments.

Be specific. To change your behavior, it is also important to be specific—when are you going to do something, how are you going to do it, with whom are you going to do it? When you are vague, you tend to fail. Writing down your intentions is very helpful; it adds to your sense of commitment. Remember that you may have to fight a tendency to avoid troublesome problems. In the short term it is all too easy to do nothing. But doing nothing will make most problems worse.

When you declare your intention to do something, that is as good as taking the first step, just as the old saying puts it: "Once begun, it's half done."

EXERCISE 11.3: PROBLEM-SOLVING ACTIONS

Now, pick up your journal again and prepare to write about the actions you will take to solve your problem and deal with the stress it has caused you. Open the journal to two blank facing pages and begin to work on the top of the left-hand page. As previously, you can write as much or as little as you choose. At the top of the page write "The solution I am working on is_____." Try to describe your solution in one or two sentences.

Your first step will be to answer the following questions:

- What resources do I need to carry out this step?

- What information do I need to carry out this step?

- Who can help to provide me with the resources and information I may need?

- What obstacles are involved in this step?

When you have answered these questions to your satisfaction, then write the following in your journal:

- I will do this step on (date and time): _____

Of course, once you've written all this down, there is a very important step that is not paper-based. That is, of course, taking all those action steps and just doing it! Once you've followed up on your plans, carry on by looking at the next section on evaluating how things went for you.

Continuous Quality Improvement (CQI)

Continuous quality improvement (CQI) is a buzzword for "planning to do better and better" in all kinds of settings, such as business, academia, and government. Problem solving also needs some CQI from time to time. It's important to know if your problem-solving attempts really did, in fact, solve the problem you had.

Once you've had the opportunity to work through the steps you plan to follow, take a moment and ask yourself, "Is my problem still here?" "Has my problem gone entirely?" "What, if anything, is still unresolved?" The term CQI was invented for organizations because most things we do are complex, and the more complicated an organization or business is, the less likely it is to run smoothly. The other parts of our lives have the same features that organizations do. Lots of things change every day that we must keep up with and manage. Many problems are not static, that is, they don't stay in one place. They move, change, and grow.

For example, suppose that you were working on the problem of wanting to improve your relationship. There may be many ideas that you brainstormed to make it better—spending more time together, communicating regularly, refraining from fighting, and so forth. However, each change you introduce will alter your relationship because your partner will react to what you do. This is called a "dynamic" situation because there are a number of forces at work at the same time. Most problems will change with time and other circumstances, so it's important to stay on top of an issue and make sure that your efforts to work on your problems are effective in both the short and long term.

Summary

This chapter examines the concept of stress and explains the link between the external events that happen to us and how our bodies respond to meet those challenges. Our brain and body are equipped to handle some amount of resistance. We have important biological wiring designed to help us weather difficulties. But too much stress can wear our bodies down, literally. Stress results in significant physical changes that affect the brain and other body systems. This is linked to depression because stress puts people at risk for this disorder.

Reducing and managing stress has a big payoff mentally and physically. We can and do make choices about how we respond to the stressors in our lives. The better we cope with stress, the less likely it is that stress will lead us into illness or depression. Quieting our minds and staying in the moment, key aspects of meditation, appear to be very useful for helping us make positive choices. Perhaps the most important notion here is that old saying, "An ounce of prevention is worth a pound of cure." To the extent that we can, we need to use problem-solving skills to keep stress from being generated in the first place. Taking an active approach to dealing with stress will help to keep both your mind and body healthy and vibrant.

CHAPTER 12

Maintaining Healthy Relationships

The relationships we have with other people are a defining feature of our lives; for some of us, our relationships are synonymous with the concept of being alive. Think about the last time you were at a funeral or listened to a tribute to someone who has passed on. At those occasions, the relationships that define us are very much in evidence. They are the first things we hear about in a memorial service; we are the spouses, mothers, fathers, sons, daughters, grandparents, and friends before we are the CEO, golfer, gardener, or anything else.

For years, researchers have understood how important relationships are; in fact, they are critical to survival. It's now understood that people who have strong relationships, especially later in life, are likely to live longer (often by many years) and enjoy a better quality of life in old age (Mahoney and Restak 1999). We seem to have an innate need to be with other people, in fact, in our society, loneliness has many of the earmarks of disease. Those who are lonely are more likely to be at risk of experiencing a host of negative mental and physical symptoms.

THE CONNECTION BETWEEN RELATIONSHIPS AND THYROID PROBLEMS

Most people reading the paragraph above would probably be in complete agreement with everything I've written. Most people intuitively understand the importance of relationships. Outside of work and sleep, we spend most of our time being with and maintaining our links with the important people in our lives. So, given these facts, what's the link between the thyroid gland and relationships? To answer that, we need to ask it scientifically, which means that we need to study the relationships of people with thyroid disorders.

If thyroid disorders do have an impact on relationships, we would expect to see problems that would not be found in a similar group who don't have thyroid problems. And this is exactly the pattern that we see. Researchers have demonstrated that thyroid disorders (including hypothyroid and hyperthyroid problems) lead to worse social functioning than is typical for most people (Bianchi et al. 2004). It also seems that these problems tend to improve when the thyroid problem is treated (Elberling et al. 2004), which confirms the idea that thyroid problems lead to interpersonal problems, as opposed to the possibility that those with thyroid problems just happen to have interpersonal relationship problems. In other words, we are fairly sure that the thyroid disorders happen first, and that these disorders can and do undermine the quality of the relationships that people with these disorders have.

Judging from your own experience, you are likely to know that your mood and behavior can be affected by your thyroid problems, and you are probably aware of the strong link between depression and thyroid problems. But what does all this have to do with your relationships? That's a fair question to ask because so far the focus has been on the thyroid-depression problem as an *intrapsychic* problem. Intrapsychic means, literally, "within the mind," and the mood problems that clearly affect those with thyroid problems are, in many ways, invisible to others. The chances are good that the average depressed person looks and acts just like anyone else. As a rule, depression doesn't exhibit itself to others. But if you got to know that person a little more, would you know that he or she suffered from depression? And if so, what would that mean to you and what would it mean to your relationship with that person?

HOW MOOD PROBLEMS BECOME RELATIONSHIP PROBLEMS

About thirty years ago, researchers in mood disorders first became interested in these questions. They began by noticing that depressed people often had serious relationship problems, much like those associated with thyroid disorders. And these researchers began to wonder how depression operates to undermine relationships. Today we know there are at least two ways depression can act to damage our emotional ties with others (Bieling and Antony 2003).

First, depression changes the way that we view our relationships with others; it changes our perceptions and, to some extent, the needs we have. For example, depressed people often become needier and have a stronger desire to be with others but, at the same time, they are often disappointed by those others; they feel less loved and supported than they felt when they were not depressed.

Second, we are now sure that depressed people act in ways that are apparent to other people when the relationship is meaningful or significant, although this difference is not noticed in more short-term interactions. The key issue is familiarity; differences aren't obvious in short interactions, but become so during repeated interactions. Studies tell us that depressed people are seen as less interesting to socialize with, and that they are more likely to be rejected by others (Segrin 2001). So, it's true that depression changes how we are perceived by others, particularly people who know us well. Loved ones, especially, become aware of the mood changes that accompany depression: the sadness, the loss of interest in life, and sometimes the irritability.

These two things, (1) changes in the way we view relationships and (2) changes in the way others see us when we are depressed, can come together in a kind of vicious cycle. Depressed people, already feeling blue and concerned about whether they will be rejected, seek reassurance from others. And, at first, those others may respond positively and reaffirm their commitment to the relationship or show their support for the depressed person in other ways. But of course, this supportiveness will not be enough to "undo" the other person's depression.

In fact, as time goes by, supporters of the depressed person begin to believe their efforts are failing, and they become frustrated because the depressed person doesn't change, and even may be asking for more reassurance. At that moment, they arrive at an important turning point. The supporters of the depressed person give up, and may even want to reduce or avoid contact with the depressed person.

So we arrive at the end of the full cycle: a depressed person who doesn't feel supported, and that person's loved ones who feel helpless and have a growing sense that living with the depressed person is hard work. The depressed person and those around him or her end up with valid concerns. This is a difficult set of circumstances to try to improve. In fact, researchers and psychologists believe that these kinds of problems help to maintain the depression and have the potential to wreak havoc in the depressed person's life.

DEPRESSION: ITS EFFECTS ON MARRIAGE

Perhaps the most significant relationship that is frequently impacted by depression is marriage. Because of the issues described above, a couple with one depressed partner is vulnerable to a deteriorating relationship. Sometimes, this gets to the point where both partners question whether they ought to remain married—many patients tell us that their marriage is "not what it used to be," that their spouse is "not the man (or woman) they married." They also say, "We've tried everything." So, in a sense, an episode of depression can end up triggering a divorce, which is one of the most stressful events in modern life. In fact, the experience of divorce can and often does trigger an episode of depression even in those who do not have mood disorders.

So the bottom line is this: Problems stemming from depression can have a devastating impact on your most important relationships. In this chapter, we hope to offer you some ways in which to do damage control when mood problems have become a part of your life. But first it's important to understand more about what happens in the relationships of depressed people, and then move on to what can be done to help matters in these circumstances.

THE RISK OF "ERODING" RELATIONSHIPS

To tackle any problem, we first have to disentangle various parts of the relationship into more reasonably sized chunks and then tackle each one bit by bit. Luckily, psychologists have been studying the relationships of depressed people for a long time and their work will help us to be more exacting in terms of where we need to focus our attention (Bieling and Antony 2003). One overarching fact is that depression appears to have an "eroding" effect on relationships (Joiner 2000).

Erosion is usually discussed in terms of geography and geology, for example, a small mountain stream that over eons creates a valley by cutting away great swathes of earth and rock, bit by bit. That is an interesting metaphor for how depression impacts relationships; in fact, it's almost a perfect metaphor. A small stream can seem to be quite placid and nonthreatening, until you look around and see how that little "trickle" has carved out the deep rent in the earth. So, too, depression at first might seem like an illness that affects only the sufferer, especially in the early stages of the disorder when loved ones often are very sympathetic.

And yet, as with the stream, people who have lived through a depression often come out on the other side, look around, and discover that their mood problem has undercut and eroded their most important supportive relationships. So it is quite important to make sure you take your depression seriously and try to prevent the usual harm that it causes to relationships.

Before moving on, let's turn back briefly to the concept of erosion: think again of watching a stream in a valley. Would you see erosion taking place? Probably not, because the process takes a lot of time to become visible to the naked eye. But if you looked closely enough, you would see soil particles being washed away, earth being churned up, small branches and leaves floating by. This process is quite subtle. So, too, with depression and relationships; the process of erosion is not easily observed. Most of the processes described below often go unnoticed, especially by the person who is depressed. In fact, these processes can become largely automatic because they are an organic part of being depressed. They are like bad habits. And, as with bad habits, there are steps to shake off these depressed processes.

- First, you have to recognize what it is you are doing.

- Second, you must really understand why that action is a problem for you.

- Third, you must be motivated to do something about the habit.

- Fourth, you have to come up with a reasonable alternative.

■ Finally, you have to follow up on that alternative and see if it works for you.

Take smoking, for example. To kick that very difficult and addictive habit you'd first have to acknowledge that you are, in truth, a compulsive smoker. Then you'd need information about how dangerous smoking is and, in order to quit, you'd really have to acknowledge that the danger is real for you, instead of denying it (known as the "It won't happen to me" syndrome). All that would become your motivation to try to quit. For most people, different kinds of support would be needed, for example, attending smoking cessation workshops and/or taking smoking cessation medications, or wearing a nicotine patch. These solutions offer alternatives for the more dangerous habit. And all of these would come to nothing unless you followed through on your commitment to attend the programs faithfully and take your medications as prescribed.

So in the remainder of this chapter I'll follow this pattern too. First, I'll describe a relationship issue that can arise during a depression so you'll be able to recognize whether it (or something like it) is happening to you. Second, I'll explain why it is a problem. Then I'll describe an alternative you can try that, hopefully, will meet your needs and not cause problems. The only thing I cannot supply is the motivation, which must come from within you, when you are ready to address these issues.

OVERVIEW OF FOUR PROBLEM AREAS

First, let's examine four very relevant areas. However, it's important to point out here that not all of these factors come into play for every depressed person. In fact, the way that depression alters relationships has a great deal to do with someone's personality before that person became depressed. That is, in some ways depression causes vulnerabilities to emerge and rise to the surface. For example, someone who thinks he is not especially attractive when he is feeling well will be likely to feel downright ugly when he is feeling depressed.

Also, over time, different combinations of these four problems may arise or they may affect several different relationships at the same time, especially when depressive episodes are long-lasting. So, be sure to look at each area carefully even if, at first, it seems to be unimportant to your situation. You may still find some relevance for your particular set of circumstances, and, more importantly, find some useful solutions.

The Four Important Problem Areas

The four major problem areas that affect the relationships of depressed people are:

1. **Dependency and reassurance-seeking:** This occurs when depressed people feel the need to really lean on others, and they believe that they can't cope alone. Often, they may fear being abandoned. Associated with this sense of "neediness" is the specific behavior of frequent checking on how others feel about them. A depressed person may ask, repeatedly, whether the other people in his life still like, love, and respect him.

2. **Irritability and distancing:** Some depressed people find that when they are down, being around other people is a source of irritation. They don't want to be bothered, believing that others' needs will be draining and overwhelming and, with their limited energy, they don't believe they can offer as much to other people as they used to. Quite often depressed people view themselves as having limited energy and patience, and they may start feeling that they don't have enough energy to keep up a social "act"; even listening to other people talking can be perceived as stressful. As a result, the depressed person may become irritable or even openly critical, rejecting, and hurtful of others.

3. **Unreasonable expectations:** Depressed people may feel they aren't getting their needs met by the others in their lives. They may experience a fairly constant sense of disappointment expressed as "Everyone is letting me down." This can lead the others in their lives to turn against them, because the depressed person's requests may come to be seen as unreasonable and unfair.

4. **Nonassertiveness and conflict avoidance:** Sometimes, depressed people tend to ignore their own needs. They don't ask for the things they want and need from others. They may fear that the others will say no to their requests. Or they may

be afraid of getting into a conflict that could add to their already depressed mood. This puts the depressed person in a difficult position in which he or she doesn't really get a "fair deal." They may feel they are putting more into relationships than they get back.

You may recognize parts of yourself when you are depressed even from these brief descriptions. Remember that these four categories do have some overlap; I've presented them this way just to keep the issues clear. People can experience these kinds of problems in combinations; for example, some people go through cycles of needing other people too much, and wanting to distance themselves from others, too. In fact, each episode of depression might create different kinds of problems within the same person.

Another factor that can be very important is the stage of the relationship. For example, if you are depressed and have just begun a new romantic relationship, the kinds of experiences you have will be quite different than if you had been married to that person for ten years and had the same episode of depression. Also, relationship dynamics can become extremely complicated. There are always two (or more) people involved and so matters can get fairly challenging. I've put together some general guidelines for dealing with these issues in the next sections, but this is an area in which professional guidance (e.g., a marriage counselor) can be a very wise choice to help you sort out what is happening.

DEPENDENCY AND REASSURANCE-SEEKING

Dependency and reassurance-seeking represent the most well-studied phenomena in depression (Bieling and Antony 2003). Nevertheless, the causes for dependency remain very complicated. What is clear is that many depressed people begin to fear, as an integral part of their depression, that they are not likeable. So they try to keep others as close to them as possible. Depressed people may come to doubt their own abilities to get things done. Those who, prior to their depression, were quite able to do things alone and make their own decisions may begin to doubt whether they can handle things without advice. Having someone beside them offering help and advice seems to make depressed people feel better.

The net result is that depressed people become intensely focused on maintaining their relationships with others, and ensuring that others are always available. Thus, depressed people turn to others, asking for their love and support, and above all checking-in to make sure the others still love them and care as much as they used to care. Reassurance-seeking can range from repeatedly asking other people's advice, to repetitive requests about the other's feelings, literally asking, "Do you still love me?" (or using similar words).

Why Reassurance-Seeking Is a Problem

At first, reassurance-seeking seems like a normal part of our relationships. Isn't it okay and perfectly normal, sometimes, to want other people to reassure us? To make sure they still care for us and want to be with us? The answer is yes, certainly, reassurance-seeking is a part of what we do in relationships, and it serves an important function; it allows us to check on the health of our relationships, and it communicates "I care about you caring about me" and "I need you." So, a relationship, especially an intimate one, in which there is no reassurance-seeking would be quite unusual, perhaps even unhealthy. But when reassurance-seeking is overdone, it is clearly very distasteful to those who are questioned.

In fact, repeated requests for reassurance may be the most repugnant behavior that depressed people practice in their relationships with others. Psychologists believe that reassurance-seeking is, simply put, the number one reason depressed people are rejected by others (Joiner 2000). But why is reassurance-seeking such a problem? This is hard to answer, except to say there is something exhausting and debilitating about having to explain, and reexplain, that we do love or care for someone. It is difficult for people to be needed too much; intense need puts too much pressure and responsibility on a person.

Moreover, there is something important in the idea of "always leave them wanting more." Social psychologists believe that we like people better when they make themselves just a little bit scarce. I don't mean unavailable or aloof, but when someone is constantly pursued by another, it's likely that the pursuer becomes less interesting to the pursued.

Also, there is the issue of repetition. Being asked once whether you still like a person might be fine, twice could also be okay, maybe even three times. But what if you asked the same question every time you saw the other person? And no matter what you said to be reassuring, it never was enough? You'd start to feel frustrated, you might think the person had never listened to your earlier answers, and that there was no way to satisfy him or her. And that is aversive; it saps your energy in ways that just spending fun time together does not. Constant reassurance-seeking can have a really bad outcome. It can lead to being rejected.

What You Can Do About Reassurance-Seeking

Obviously, the reason for presenting this information about reassurance-seeking is to make you aware of what it is and what it does. In order for anyone to change his or her behavior, to do something differently, that person needs to know what it is they are doing ("How can I recognize it?") and why it is a problem ("Why I should do something about it."). So, now you know why reassurance-seeking is a problem and why you should do something about it. The bottom line is the number of times you engage in reassurance-seeking should be as few as possible.

Unfortunately, asking for reassurance is likely to become slightly automatic as a response to being depressed. The need to ask for reassurance might just sneak up on you and take place before you know it's happening. So, it's important to become sensitive to your need for reassurance, and the first place you'll notice this is in your thinking and feeling. Remember in chapter 10 I described the connection between depression and negative, self-defeating thinking? This is important here, too, because *people ask for reassurance when they have doubts about the other person's feelings or commitment toward them.* Reassurance-seeking is supposed to put those doubts to rest, which in the long run it doesn't actually do.

So, before you ask for reassurance, you might notice you have certain kinds of thoughts like, "Can I really count on this person?" "Does he/she care about me the way they used to?" "I'm not sure he/she has been as attentive to me as usual." A real list could be much longer, but the thoughts have similar themes; they represent your worry about the connection you have with someone else.

But this is the place where you have an opportunity to catch yourself and to notice what you are thinking. This is the place to recognize that your thoughts might be your depressed brain telling you a story, and, probably, a false one. Before you seek reassurance, slow down and check out whether there is any truth to your thoughts. What is your real evidence that the other person has changed? Are the changes just part of everyday events, or are they signs of rejection? What are the costs of asking for reassurance all the time? Indeed, depressed people sometimes don't even recognize that asking for reassurance has any costs, and it clearly does.

Finally, it is most likely inevitable that you will ask for reassurance sometimes, and remember that some amount of checking-in is normal in any relationship. So, if you find yourself asking the question "Do you still like me the way you used to?" do yourself a favor and really listen to the answer. Part of what causes excessive reassurance-seeking is that the depressed person is waiting for a completely satisfying answer.

Depressed people are, in fact, prone to identifying flaws in the answer they get (e.g., the person told me he/she loved me only because I asked, he/she left out something I was looking for in the answer). This, too, is more than likely to be the product of the depressed person's way of thinking, and, of course, it makes it more likely that the person will go fishing later for another kind of answer. So make sure that when you ask a question, you appreciate the answer and not be too critical of what you hear.

IRRITABILITY AND DISTANCING

Just as some depressed people find themselves drawn to others for reassurance that the relationship is still strong, depression can result in withdrawing socially and feeling the need for isolation—sometimes even becoming irritated with other people (Bieling and Alden 2001; Blatt and Zuroff 1992). Some people experience a mixture of alternating periods of needing others followed by periods of irritation with others. This irritability and need to put distance between oneself and others is based on two kinds of beliefs.

First, that other people are a drain on the depressed person's very limited energy. Second, that other people have expectations, which sometimes the depressed person may feel anxious about living up to.

Depressed people may have a sense that being around others requires them to be "on" in a kind of performance, part of which might be having to pretend that they are fine and act as if nothing is wrong. In the long run, because of the perceived pressure of being around others, the depressed person will try to avoid social interactions, sometimes at all costs. Even worse, when they must engage in interactions with others, the depressed person might signal his or her irritation and anger, in addition to being anxious.

Why Distancing and Irritability Are Problems

Of all the interpersonal problems that accompany depression, the problem of distancing is perhaps the most difficult to change. The reason for this seems to be that people who are isolating themselves (and who become irritated in social situations) are unlikely to really feel any need to be different. Their everyday experience is that they feel better when they avoid social situations, and they often become upset and worse when they interact with others. In other words, they have powerful, seemingly rational reasons for being where they are. But let's not forget, where they are is still depressed. And the benefit they gain from avoiding others is very short term. It's also important to consider what the long-terms costs are. When avoidance takes over, these costs are considerable.

First, to have a good quality of life, we need positive relationships with other people. If depressed people who are distancing and avoiding others carry on doing what seems to come naturally, their social circle will become smaller and smaller. Some people become virtually housebound. Those who reach this stage have terrible difficulties reestablishing social contacts; their anxiety levels often go through the roof when they must interact with others.

Second, this avoidance and irritability have a tremendous impact on other people. Usually, at some point, even very close friends and family will give up on those who are isolating themselves. And that may outlast the depressive episode, which can be very sad. So, even if depressed people eventually recover (by whatever means), they are still left to deal with social relationships in which their friends and relatives feel hurt and rejected. The other people in the lives of depressed people already have trouble understanding what depression is and how to respond to it. But when the depression is accompanied by a great deal of avoidance and irritability, the social costs can be huge.

No doubt this is partly due to the stigma that surrounds mental illness, where even the victim can be blamed because other people may have little sympathy for what it's like to be depressed. But we also must live in the world as it is, not as it should be; and so it can be critical to try to maintain your relationships and to help them survive through difficult times.

None of the information provided here is designed to frighten depressed people into changing their patterns of distancing and avoidance, but the material is honest and up front. In the long run, considering the real-world consequences of your actions is very motivational. Such thought can help you to resist the urge to give into more short-term satisfaction, which often seems like the easier way to go.

What You Can Do About Distancing and Avoidance

There are two parts for dealing with this issue in a proactive way, both of which have to do with keeping the lines of communication open. First, it's important to examine your beliefs about what other people expect of you. Second, it'll be important to refocus your attention and effort on what it is you get out of your relationships.

Others' expectations. It is quite difficult to be social when we perceive that we need to act or be a certain way. This can make us feel as if there is a spotlight on us, that every nuance of our behavior is being looked at and judged. When depressed, it is difficult to have the energy and motivation to appear happy, and often this can lead to difficulties. Indeed "acting normal" is, probably, impossible. Trying to act not depressed, that is, trying to act like your usual self, would present an insurmountable challenge. So, if this is the standard you are applying to yourself, consciously or perhaps not so consciously, it wouldn't be surprising if you find yourself dreading being with other people.

So, to reduce your avoidance and irritation with others, it's important to acknowledge your limitations; not to others, but to yourself. But should you tell other people that you are depressed? This is an important topic in and of itself. Stigma-busting is an important thing to do, and, of course, you have the right to tell anyone you want to about your depression, perhaps even provide them with some education. But because some people will be judgmental, you should be aware that you might not always like the consequences of revealing that you are depressed. Certainly, very close family and friends probably do need to be told what is going on. However, for other social relationships, it may not be necessary to explain that you are depressed.

After reviewing the next section on assertiveness, however, what you probably do want to communicate is what your needs are and what you can handle socially right now. Even if other people notice that you are not your usual self, there will be no surprises. When people know what to expect of you, they are likely to be more understanding, and you will feel less pressure and more ability to socialize.

Your social needs. Remembering that being with other people is not meant to be energy-draining is equally important. But depression often leads to this perception. It's as if every social obligation is just that, something that you have to go to, where you will be required to spend your energy but you feel that nothing is returned to you. In order to maintain social connections, there has to be something in it for you too. When we are not depressed, this process is natural enough. We enjoy the conversation, advice, story-sharing, perhaps just feeling connected with other people. During an episode of depression, however, it can also be important to figure out what you need to get from being with others. One of the most difficult aspects of being depressed is that people lose the sense of being in control of their own destiny. In that sense, being with other people can be somewhat frightening and off-putting.

There is almost a fear that we won't be able to say no when we need to, and that other people may even take advantage of us. Being able to say no is part of being assertive, which is discussed later in this chapter. But, as your first priority, you must know what it is you want from whatever social interactions you enter. Remember that having positive social interactions is a huge part of recovering from depression.

Even while you are depressed, it's important to choose to participate in some social interactions. One way to get some control over these interactions is to issue invitations yourself as much as possible. For example, you could ask a friend to go with you to a movie or concert. That way, you can have more say over what you will be doing, for how long, with whom, and so forth. The bottom line is that avoiding social interactions will make it more difficult for you to recover, and engaging in meaningful social interactions will lead to important improvements.

UNREASONABLE EXPECTATIONS

Among all the challenges that depression creates for relationships, the expectations that we have for others is one of the most subtle and insidious. Briefly, just as someone who is depressed tends to view all events through a negative lens (like a dark set of sunglasses), so, too, relationships are often scrutinized in a similar, quite often critical, manner. For some depressed people, their negative thoughts will focus on a nagging feeling of disappointment, of being constantly let down, most often with close relationships like marriage or in the immediate family. But when these kinds of judgments are made, they are probably related to the symptoms of depression, especially when the depressed people try to find an explanation for why they feel so down. This seems to be part of our natural, human tendency to seek explanations for our feelings. If I am feeling down, it makes sense for me to ask, "Why am I so down?" or "What is happening in my life that might be causing these bad feelings?" Sometimes, rather than acknowledge an illness is at work, depressed people will focus on other factors, perhaps ending up believing that a problem in a relationship leads to all their distress. This can start a cycle in which depressed people scrutinize their relationships for problems and then become highly sensitive to any perceived shortcomings.

Why Unreasonable Expectations Are a Problem

High expectations followed by disappointment can result in a number of difficulties. First, depressed people may not properly recognize that they do have an illness, that is, they are depressed. They may come to believe that a relationship is causing all of their problems. Most often, the relationship that becomes the focus of their concern, perhaps unfairly, is their marriage. This belief can result in their depression not being treated properly. For example, depressed people may not take their antidepressant medication because they may believe, very strongly, that what they really need is marital therapy, or worse, to leave the marriage. I have seen cases in which depressed people sought and obtained divorces, only to realize that their mood is even worse afterward.

Second, high expectations can be very hard on the other person in a relationship; they can cause the person who loves you to wonder desperately about what else he or she can do to help you. Eventually, their frustration will grow to the point where they, too, lash out, or they withdraw because they know they can't live up to your expectations.

The most frustrating aspect of this process is that, if left unchecked, a relationship that was just fine gets labeled as a problem. That labeling in and of itself can serve to undermine the relationship, to the point where a real problem is created. Sadly, too, some of these relationships will end when, in a very real way, there were no problems prior to the depression.

What You Can Do About Unreasonable Expectations

Many of the strategies described in chapter 10, all of which can help you to analyze your thoughts more rationally and objectively, will be helpful when applied to your relationships. The most basic and important question to ask yourself is this: "Are my expectations reasonable and fair?" Do you want the people in your life to do too much? Are they being asked to give you more than they are getting back, more than they are capable of? More than you expected of them before you became depressed? Of course, when you are depressed, inevitably, you will have different needs. It is fine to express those, just as is described in the next section. The difficulty comes from balancing your needs and expectations with those of the people you love and who you want to love and support you. For relationships to work, they must be two-way streets; in the long run we need to give and get back in equal portions.

One other very important thing to remember is to move very cautiously when it comes to important relationships. So often, when people feel they are not getting what they need, they make rash decisions. In depression, the most profound of these rash decisions is to leave a marriage or an intimate relationship. It used to be common in some forms of therapy that the client made a commitment not to change anything drastic about their lives while in treatment, that is, like getting married or divorced, or changing careers. Although nothing should be seen as an absolute, the idea behind this is probably still sound; do not make permanent decisions for yourself unless and until your mind and emotions are very clear and stable. Otherwise, you may be responding to your symptoms, and not to your long-run needs and your own best interests. Of course, when you do find that your expectations are indeed both reasonable and unmet, the next section on nonassertiveness will be most helpful.

NONASSERTIVENESS AND CONFLICT AVOIDANCE

The difficulty with nonassertiveness may be easier to understand, but no less problematic if left unchecked. Essentially, assertiveness can be defined as two things: (1) asking for your needs to be met, and (2) refusing requests that seem unreasonable to you. There is a difference between being too assertive and being aggressive. With assertiveness, we respect other people's opinions and understand that other people have every right to say no. (Remember that your request to have your needs met may conflict with another person's need to refuse unreasonable requests.) People who are aggressive do not have this perspective; unfortunately they may have a "take no prisoners" approach to things that is very off-putting and disrespect-ful. So, assertiveness is a positive and important component of our social lives. In a depression, however, assertiveness is likely to be compromised for several reasons.

First, depressed people may lack the energy to stand up for them-selves. Second, depressed people sometimes believe their needs are not important; this can be part of the loss of self-esteem that seems to be integral to depression. The bottom line is that depressed people are unlikely to feel themselves to be in a position to ask for things they would like from others. For that reason, they sometimes may say yes to unreasonable requests, when their true answer would normally be no.

Sometimes, standing up for ourselves leads to squabbles and disagreements—that is, to conflict. But then sometimes conflict needs to happen between people to arrive at a new understanding, especially in a marriage or intimate relationship. Conflicts are never pleasant. It'd be nice to never have them, but they are part of human communica-tion; they help to reestablish equilibrium and balance in a relationship. Not being assertive probably means not ever engaging in conflict if it can be avoided.

Why Nonassertiveness Is a Problem

For someone who is depressed, nonassertiveness probably represents a slow but steady form of erosion, and it operates as a vicious cycle. In relationships, part of the give and take is to ask for what you need, and to provide the same for the other person. We cannot be satisfied or happy if other people don't meet our needs, and the only way to get our needs met is to ask. So, because others can't read our minds, if we do not ask for what we need, it is unlikely that others will provide us with what we want.

When people don't ask for their needs to be met, or are forced to make compromises when they don't want to, they are likely to feel even worse about themselves. Eventually, they will become very frustrated with their relationships. Our perceptions of the quality of most relationships have to do with whether (or not) the other person is meeting our needs. Sometimes this leads to a sudden angry snap or a lashing out. Every time our needs aren't met, a small piece of resentment gets added, because, at some level, even depressed people measure what they receive against what they put into a relationship. At some point, these people will have had enough, and their building resentment will boil over in an angry outburst, venting all of their frustration. For the other person in the relationship, this often comes as quite a surprise. They may have noticed nothing more than the fact that their partner had been very accommodating previously.

In fact, depressed people often observe that the other people they have relationships with are self-centered and ignore their needs. But when probed further, it often turns out that this is, at least in part, because the depressed person has taken a very passive approach to the relationship. Depressed people often expect others ought to know what it is they want. The fact is, for better or worse, people tend to take care of their own needs first. This is a basic right we all have. In a sense then, we are self-centered.

There is indeed a fine line between being assertive and being selfish. In fact, being self-centered is probably good for a person's mood, even when, in the extreme, it is hardly a wonderful trait. The bottom line is that we live in a world of relationships where we have things we need, and things we can provide. To have stable and good relationships we need to receive as much as we give; relationships in which one person gives more than the other are notoriously unstable. So standing up for ourselves is more than just being concerned about our needs, it's also about keeping our relationships balanced. Unbalanced relationships are neither stable nor happy.

Another important fact to consider is that when people are assertive, they can wind up in conflict. Standing up for what we want sometimes does mean negotiating or even agreeing to disagree because others may not be inclined to agree. And by the word "negotiate" I mean that when we are assertive, fighting or arguing is a possible outcome. Depressed people seem to want to avoid fights or arguments. They may fear that they are likely to lose the argument in any conflict, perhaps they also fear that by rocking the boat they risk losing the relationship.

What's important to recognize is that, to some extent, fighting and arguments measure the strength of a relationship just as much as intimacy or closeness. We can fight when we feel confident that a fight will not be the end of the world, that there will be a resolution and a future day when the difficulty has been phased out. Avoiding conflict might be desirable for someone who is depressed, but it is a short-term gain only. In the long run, not being able to engage in conflict means that your resentments will continue to grow and your needs will continue to be unmet. Being assertive does not always wind up getting you what you want, so, in that sense, assertion will not always succeed. However, there is a very real benefit to be gained by speaking your mind and asking for what you want.

What You Can Do About Assertiveness

Assertiveness is an important topic; one about which entire books have been written (e.g., Davis, Paleg, and Fanning 2004; Fleming 1997; Paterson 2000). So, here, I will provide an overview of what these books say about assertion. As usual, the first step is to understand the need for assertiveness, which I hope is clear from the preceding section. To sum that up, assertion helps to get your needs met (a plus for you) and it helps to keep a relationship balanced and stable (a real plus for the relationship). Next I will provide some general guidelines for making requests to have your needs met, followed by some advice on how to say no assertively.

Fundamentally, being assertive is about communicating your needs, i.e., saying what it is you want. This seems easy, but there are many little things that you can do to communicate your needs effectively. The main point is to position yourself somewhere between being too passive (a real risk with depression) and being overly aggressive (something that happens when resentment builds up for too long). The most common error that occurs when people are learning to be more assertive is either they are not quite clear enough (too passive) or they ask for their needs while, at the same time, they step on someone else's rights or feelings (too aggressive).

So to avoid these mistakes, it's important to get used to communicating assertively by following a certain kind of pattern with three distinct steps. These are:

1. **Summarize your position.** Describe your perceptions of a situation, what you think is happening, what you think is the bottom line.

2. **Describe how you feel.** Tell the other person how the situation (as you see it) is affecting your emotional life so he or she will know the situation matters to you.

3. **Ask for what you want.** Focus on solutions. What could make this better for you? What could the other person do to soothe the situation and the feelings you have?

To have an honest communication, each step is equally important, as is allowing the other person to respond. Notice that you are not only making the other person aware of a problem, but pointing a way to a solution by saying what it is you want. This is as large a part of effective assertion as describing what the problem is.

Sometimes, people planning to be assertive will experience considerable anxiety about asking for what they want, especially if they usually put off asking for their needs to be met. In that case, it might be helpful to write down (or at very least plan) what you want to say. It might be helpful to actually rehearse what you want to say, even in your mind's eye, and to also consider what the other person might say in response. Will the other person be surprised by your request? Will he or she become upset or angry? What does the other person give up by agreeing to your request? Considering these options will help you to shape what you are going to say, and how you are going to say it.

Another thing to consider is how you want to come across when you are assertive because when and how you present your request might have a lot to do with determining the success of that request. When people struggle to be assertive they sometimes forget to consider some basic things that are essential to all communication. These are:

1. **Timing.** Pick a time that works for you and for the other person to have the conversation. If necessary, make an appointment to talk to that person so that he or she will have the time to discuss your request.

2. **Eye contact.** While you are not trying to stare down the other person or be threatening, a moderate level of eye contact does communicate that you are serious and stand behind whatever it is that you are saying.

3. **Tone of voice.** This too should be moderate, clear, and loud enough to be heard, but be careful not to have an edge of irritation if you can help it.

4. **Posture.** Our nonverbal behavior signals a lot about how we feel; when we are not being assertive we make ourselves seem smaller with drooping shoulders, heads bent down, and legs together. To be assertive, try a more open, dignified, and erect posture to put some body language together with your assertive words.

So, an assertive statement takes the three steps—what you see going on, how it makes you feel, and what you want to be different—and combines them with good solid communication skills in an attempt to have your needs met. You'll probably be surprised by how well these skills work, even when they don't get your needs met immediately; a channel of dialogue will have been opened that in the long run will give you more chance of succeeding.

What about the issue of saying no to unreasonable requests, the second half of being assertive? To some extent, the same skills apply here. If someone were to ask you to do something that you don't think is reasonable, or even if you simply don't want to do it, you can (1) summarize what he or she is asking for, (2) describe your feelings in response to that request, and (3) say no. Step 3 might seem obvious, but I have found that people sometimes forget to actually say this, which is not very assertive and may confuse the other person. Together, the three steps help the other person to understand that you are saying no and also why you are saying no. The communication skills (e.g., eye contact, tone of voice) for saying no are similar to the skills used when asking for something you want.

Finally, there are some well-known techniques that can be used to deal with a variety of situations, particularly situations in which some amount of conflict is present:

1. **Fogging.** This is useful when someone is criticizing you. The basic idea is to agree with the criticism, or at least accept the grain of truth in it, but still respond with the same perspective you had before the criticism was made.

2. **Broken record.** This is useful when someone is just not getting it, especially when you have turned down an unreasonable request and the other person keeps trying to convince you to change your mind. Sometimes, being asked the same request or question over and over again makes us want to find new reasons to say no, or to want to explain ourselves better. Remember that you don't have to do this; you can simply repeat the same answer you gave the first time a second, third, or fourth time. This will cause the other person to give up fairly quickly, and you'll avoid the energy drain that comes from having to think of new arguments to support your view of the matter.

3. **Praise.** Sometimes, you can disarm the other person, especially in a conflict situation, if you can find something nice to say about him or her (it should be something you truly believe or you will be seen as insincere). This helps to communicate the information that the situation has not turned you or the other person into an enemy.

4. **Redirect.** You don't always have to respond directly to the other person's argument against what you want. You can acknowledge what he or she has said but also respond with a completely different idea that is more in line with getting your needs met.

5. **Negative inquiry.** This is useful if you are being criticized, because with this strategy you ask the other person if he or she has any other criticisms of you, aside from what has already been stated. By asking this, you move past the criticism, without necessarily agreeing with it. Often, the other person will be disarmed by this "acceptance" tactic. You can

then talk about what needs to happen next, which is probably more important and more productive, too.

6. **Compromise.** If you feel your position is clear and the other person's position is also clear, instead of aiming to win (or possibly lose), ask directly whether compromise is possible. This immediately communicates that your position is a reasonable one to negotiate around. It also communicates that you are being open-minded and fair.

Communicating assertively is a skill that does include many subtleties. Like any skill, it can be learned, practiced, and you can get quite good at it. But if you don't practice, your skills will start to diminish. At their best, assertiveness skills can be very persuasive and still help you to maintain relationships that are balanced, lively, and mutually satisfying.

As a final note on assertiveness, many depressed people who made a commitment to make changes by using these skills notice two things. The first is that they experience more confrontations, sometimes even arguments, with other people. At least in part, this is due to the fact that the depressed person's friends and families have become used to the depressed person being passive, and they are somewhat taken aback by this new approach.

The second thing that these newly assertive people notice is that they get more of their needs satisfied, that they are treated with a new kind of respect, and they get a fairer deal from other people. Obviously, the second part, that is, getting more of your needs met, is a wonderful outcome. But so is shaking up the status quo, finding out that you are no longer afraid to disagree, and finding out that conflicts can be survived without any lasting damage. The change sometimes can be disconcerting, even a little difficult, but I have yet to meet a person who regretted being assertive when all was, literally, said and done.

SOME FINAL WORDS ON HEALTHY INTERPERSONAL RELATIONSHIPS

A number of themes are important to emphasize here. First, all of the problems that depression causes in relationships have to do with balance; harmonious relationships have a healthy exchange of support, love, and intimacy. Relationships in which one person does more of the heavy lifting rarely last. Second, depression undermines good communication. Somehow, expectations, needs, and wants do not get communicated and are therefore at risk of not being met. When people don't know what it is they want, the others in their lives can't provide it for them. At the same time, what you ask for must be fair and reasonable. We are happy when we have good relationships, but relationships alone cannot always provide us with a good mood.

Relationships also can be very complex, and one chapter in a book like this may not be enough to solve deep problems that have been ongoing for a while. Marriage is often the most vexing and complicated relationship affected negatively by depression. And sometimes marital problems, especially those that arrive prior to a major mood shift, can trigger a depression. This is when the advice of a professional can be the most helpful. Marital therapy can be very helpful for sorting out what the problems are. A well-trained professional can be invaluable in diagnosing what is going on in a relationship. Such an expert observer will have an objective view of your situation, and will see things that you yourself may not.

Interpersonal therapy. There is a specific treatment for depression called interpersonal therapy (or IPT) that has proven itself to be very effective; it can do as much for symptoms of depression as antidepressants do. IPT, as its name implies, focuses specifically on relationships. Unfortunately, it is too difficult to describe IPT properly in just one chapter. To learn more, read *Mastering Depression Through Interpersonal Psychotherapy: Patient Workbook* by Myrna Weissman (2000), a founder of the approach. This book will provide you with much more detail about how to use IPT to overcome problems with depression. To orient you to this approach, a brief overview is offered below.

FOUR AREAS OF FOCUS

One way to find out if IPT is for you is to learn a little about the treatment. When people visit an IPT therapist, they will work on one of four different areas, usually the one that is causing the most problems.

1. **Grief.** This area concerns the death of a loved one, and all the associated losses we experience when someone close to us passes away. Therapy focused on grief involves discussing your emotional responses to the loss, and acknowledging all

the ways in which the lost relationship had meaning for you and contributed to your life. And then finding a way to meet those needs in another way, or from another relationship.

2. **Interpersonal role disputes.** This area usually involves disagreements between what you would like to have in a relationship and what others would like to have from you. So, in light of the previous discussion, if you have been assertive and asked for your needs to be met, and someone else has communicated that he or she is not prepared to meet those needs, basically, you are in an interpersonal role dispute. Working out these differences, which often can end up as a standoff, or deadlocked tie, can require some expert advice. Negotiation and compromise are likely to be part of the answer for this kind of problem.

3. **Role transitions.** This area involves life changes that require taking on new kinds of tasks and demands, and possibly giving up other things that someone might regret giving up. Often, these transitions happen as a result of life changes like getting married, having a child, or retiring. When these important events take place, often we are forced to follow a certain kind of script, or role. For example, when people make the transition from being single to being married, their time is no longer their own to spend as they please. In addition to their time, their resources may also have to be shared all the time. There may be other changes they don't expect, and new ways of behaving that don't really suit them. They may have to give up some things that were previously enjoyed, like spending time alone. People may feel as if they are out of step with what they should be doing. They may have regrets and wish that things were the way they used to be. Using IPT for role transitions can help to make you more comfortable while you are settling into your new role. It can also show you how to cope better with some of the things you may have had to give up in your new role.

4. **Interpersonal skills.** There is probably more complexity in relationships than just about any other area of psychology that matters to our health and well-being. And there are many communication skills that apply to making lasting and

satisfying relationships. Using IPT to improve their skills helps people to look at whatever shortcomings they are currently experiencing in their relationships and helps to coach them in developing those skills.

Summary

Relationships are always at risk when we are depressed. A serious depression changes us in ways that are probably as obvious to others as they are to ourselves. More than that, depression can cause serious problems in communication that, if left unchecked, can quickly undermine our relationships so that we begin to lose the very valuable social support and social contact we all need.

Communicating is a complex business. I've tried to provide a brief overview of the most obvious problems that occur with a depression and some fixes to help those problems. There are other excellent resources to help people with communication; one the best resources my patients have found is a book called *Messages* by McKay, Davis, and Fanning (1995). There is also an excellent workbook that goes with that book (Davis, Paleg, and Fanning, 2004). Also, Deborah Tannen has written several excellent books on communication patterns, both for relationships in general (1991) and for relationships between men and women (2001). Keeping the lines of communication open is the best thing you can do for your relationships, and getting professional help to do this may be important too.

References

Agid, O., and B. Lerer. 2003. Algorithm-based treatment of major depression in an outpatient clinic: Clinical correlates of response to a specific serotonin reuptake inhibitor and to triiodothyronine augmentation. *International Journal of Neuropsychopharmacology* 6(1):41-49.

American Psychiatric Association. 1994. *Diagnostic and Statistical Manual of Mental Disorders*. 4th ed. Washington, DC: American Psychiatric Association.

Arem, R. 1999a. Stress and thyroid imbalance: Which comes first? In *The Thyroid Solution: A Mind-Body Program for Beating Depression and Regaining Your Emotional and Physical Health*. Edited by A. Gold. New York: Ballantine Books.

Arem, R. 1999b. Thyroid imbalance, depression, anxiety, and mood swings. In *The Thyroid Solution: A Mind-Body Program for Beating Depression and Regaining Your Emotional and Physical Health*. Edited by A. Gold. New York: Ballantine Books.

Arem, R. 1999c. Medicine from the body: thyroid hormone as an antidepressant. In *The Thyroid Solution: A Mind-Body Program for Beating Depression and Regaining Your Emotional and Physical Health*. Edited by A. Gold. New York: Ballantine Books.

Ashner, R. 1949. Myxedematous madness. *British Medical Journal* 2:555.

Barnes, B. O. 1976. The thyroid in emotional and behavioral problems. In *Hypothyroidism: The Unsuspected Illness*. New York: Harper & Row.

Beck, A. T. 1967. *Depression: Clinical, Experimental, and Theoretical Aspects.* New York: Harper & Row.

Bianchi, G. P., V. Zaccheroni, E. Solarli, F. Vescini, R. Cerutti, M. Zoli, et al. 2004. Health-related quality of life in patients with thyroid disorders. *Quality of Life Research* 13:45-54.

Bieling, P. J., and L. E. Alden. 2001. Sociotropy, autonomy, and the interpersonal model of depression: An integration. *Cognitive Therapy and Research* 25:167-184.

Bieling, P. J., and M. M. Antony. 2003. *Ending the Depression Cycle.* Oakland, CA: New Harbinger Publications.

Billings, A. G., R. C. Cronkite, and R. H. Moos. 1983. Social-environmental factors in unipolar depression: Comparisons of depressed patients and nondepressed controls. *Journal of Abnormal Psychology* 92:119-133.

Blatt, S. J., and D. C. Zuroff. 1992. Interpersonal relatedness and self-definition: Two prototypes for depression. *Clinical Psychology Review* 12:527-562.

Bootzin, R. R., and S. P. Rider. 1997. Behavioral techniques and biofeedback for insomnia. In *Understanding Sleep: The Evaluation and Treatment of Sleep Disorders.* Edited by M. R. Pressman and W. C. Orr. Washington, DC: American Psychological Association.

Braam, A. W., P. van den Eeden, M. J. Prince, A. T. F. Beekman, S. L. Kivelä, B. A. Lawlor, et al. 2001. Religion as a cross-cultural determinant of depression in elderly Europeans: Results from the EURODEP collaboration. *Psychological Medicine* 31:803-814.

Brosse, A. L., E. S. Sheets, H. S. Lett, and J. A. Blumenthal. 2002. Exercise and the treatment of clinical depression in adults: Recent findings and future directions. *Sports Medicine* 32:741-760.

Brownstein, D. 2002. *Overcoming Thyroid Disorders.* West Bloomfield, MI: Medical Alternatives Press.

Burns, D. D. 1999. *The Feeling Good Handbook.* Rev. ed. New York: Plume.

Clark, D. A., A. T. Beck, with B. A. Alford. 1999. *Scientific Foundations of Cognitive Theory and Therapy of Depression.* Chichester, UK: Wiley & Sons.

Coren, S. 1996. *Sleep Thieves: An Eye-Opening Exploration into the Science and Mysteries of Sleep.* New York: Free Press.

Costa, E., and J. Silva. 2005. Overview of the field. *Metabolism* 54(5):S5-S9.

Cotman, C. W., and N. C. Berchtold. 2002. Exercise: A behavioral intervention to enhance brain health and plasticity. *Trends in Neurosciences* 25:295-301.

Cronkite, R. C., and R. H. Moos. 1995. Life context, coping strategies, and depression. In *Handbook of Depression*. 2nd. ed. Edited by E. E. Beckham and W. R. Leber. New York: Guilford Press.

Davis, M., K. Paleg, and P. Fanning. 2004. *The Messages Workbook: Powerful Strategies for Effective Communication at Work and Home*. Oakland, CA: New Harbinger Publications.

Dratman, M. B., and J. T. Gordon. 1996. Thyroid hormones as neurotransmitters. *Thyroid* 6(6):639-647.

Dunn, A. L., M. H. Trivedi, J. B. Kampert, C. G. Clark, and H. O. Chambliss. 2005. Exercise treatment for depression: Efficacy and dose response. *American Journal of Preventive Medicine* 28:1-8.

Elberling, T. V., A. K. Rasmussen, U. Feldt-Rasmussen, M. Hording, H. Perrild, and G. Waldemar. 2004. Impaired health-related quality of life in Graves' disease: A prospective study. *European Journal of Endocrinology* 151:549-555.

Fester, C. B. 1973. A functional analysis of depression. *American Psychologist* 28:857-870.

Fleming, J. 1997. *Become Assertive!* Kent, UK: David Grant Publishing.

Fountoulakis, K. N., A. Iacovides, P. Grammaticos, G. St. Kaprinis, and P. Bech. 2004. Thyroid function in clinical subtypes of major depression: An exploratory study. *BMC Psychiatry* 4(1):6.

Frankl, V. 1959. *Man's Search for Meaning*. Boston: Beacon Press.

Fukao, A., J. Takamatsu, Y. Murakami, S. Sakane, A. Miyauchi, K. Kuma, et al. 2003. The relationship of psychological factors to the prognosis of hyperthyroidism in antithyroid drug-treated patients with Graves' disease. *Clinical Endocrinology* 58:550-555.

Gaby, A. R. 2003. Hypothyroidism: Notes. In *Nutritional Therapy in Medical Practice*. Carlisle, PA: Nutrition Seminars.

Gold, M., S. Pottash, and A. L. C. Extein. 1982. "Symptomless" autoimmune thyroiditis in depression. *Psychiatry Research* 6:261-269.

Goldapple, K., Z. Segal, C. Garson, M. Lau, P. J. Bieling, S. Kennedy, et al. 2004. Modulation of cortical-limbic pathways in major depression: Treatment specific effects of cognitive behavioral therapy. *Archives of General Psychiatry* 61:34-41.

Gortner, E. T., J. K. Gollan, K. S. Dobson, and N. S. Jacobson. 1998. Cognitive-behavioral treatment for depression: Relapse prevention. *Journal of Consulting and Clinical Psychology* 66:377-384.

Greenberger, D., and C. A. Padesky. 1995. *Mind Over Mood: How to Change the Way You Feel by Changing the Way You Think*. New York: Guilford Press.

Haggerty, J. J., Jr., R. A. Stern, G. A. Mason, J. Beckwith, C. E. Morey, and A. J. Prange Jr. 1993. Subclinical hypothyroidism: A modifiable risk factor for depression? *American Journal of Psychiatry* 150:508-510.

Hayes, S. C., K. D. Strosahl, and K. G. Wilson. 1999. *Acceptance and Commitment Therapy: An Experiential Approach to Behavior Change.* New York: Guilford Press.

Hendrick, V., L. Altshuler, and G. Whybrow. 1998. Psychoneuroendocrinology of mood disorders. *Psychiatric Clinics of North America* 21(2):277-292.

Henley, W., and N. Koehnle. 1997. Thyroid hormones and the treatment of depression: An examination of basic hormonal actions in the mature mammalian brain. *Synapse* 27:36-44.

Hofstetter, J. R., P. H. Lysaker, and A. R. Mayeda. 2005. Quality of sleep in patients with schizophrenia is associated with quality of life and coping. *BMC Psychiatry* 5:13.

Jacobson, N. S., K. S. Dobson, P. A. Truax, M. E. Addis, K. Koerner, J. K. Gollan, et al. 1996. A component analysis of cognitive-behavioral treatment for depression. *Journal of Consulting and Clinical Psychology* 64:295-304.

Joffe, R. T. 2002. Psychopharmacology for the clinician. *Journal of Psychiatry and Neuroscience* 27(1):80.

Joffe, R. T., Z. Segal, and W. Singer. 1996. Change in thyroid hormone levels following response to cognitive therapy for major depression. *American Journal of Psychiatry* 153:411-413.

Joffe, R. T., S. T. Sokolov, and W. Singer. 1995. Thyroid hormone treatment of depression. *Thyroid* 5(3):235-239.

Joiner, T. E. 2000. Depression's vicious scree: Self-propagating and erosive processes in depression chronicity. *Clinical Psychology Science and Practice* 7:203-218.

Kabat-Zinn, J. 1990. *Full Catastrophe Living: Using the Wisdom of Your Body and Mind to Face Stress, Pain, and Illness.* New York: Dell Publishing.

Kelly, G. S. 2000. Peripheral metabolism of thyroid hormones. *Alternative Medicine Review* 5(4):306-330.

Kirkegaard, C., and J. Faber. 1998. The role of thyroid hormones in depression. *European Journal of Endocrinology* 138:1-9.

Koenig, H. G., D. B. Larson, and S. S. Larson. 2001. Religion and coping with serious medical illness. *Annals of Pharmacotherapy* 35:352-359.

Kralik, A., K. Eder, and M. Kirchgessner. 1996. Influence of zinc and selenium deficiency on parameters relating to thyroid hormone metabolism. *Hormone and Metabolic Research* 28:223-226.

Larsen, P. R., H. M. Kronenberg, S. Melmed, and K. S. Polansky. 2003. *Williams Textbook of Endocrinology*. 10th ed. Boston: Elsevier.

Lewinsohn, P. M. 1974. A behavioral approach to depression. In *The Psychology of Depression: Contemporary Theory and Research*. Edited by R. J. Friedman and M. M. Katz. New York: Wiley & Sons.

Mahoney, D., and R. Restak. 1999. *The Longevity Strategy: How to Live to 100 Using the Brain-Body Connection*. Toronto, ON: John Wiley & Sons Canada.

Mason, G. A., C. H. Walker, and A. J. Prange Jr. 1993. L-Triiodothyronine: Is this peripheral hormone a central neurotransmitter? *Neuropsychopharmacology* 8(3):253-258.

Mazzaferri, E. L. 1989. Thyroid function tests. *Post-Graduate Medicine* 85(5):333-352.

McEwen, B. S. 1995. Stress and neuroendocrine function: Individual differences and mechanisms leading to disease. In *Psychoneuroendocrinology: The Scientific Basis of Clinical Practice*. Edited by O. W. Wolkowitz and A. J. Rothschild. Washington, DC: American Psychiatric Publishing.

McEwen, B. S. 2003. Stressful experience, brain, and emotions: Developmental, genetic, and hormonal influences. In *The Cognitive Neurosciences*. Edited by M. S. Gazzaniga. Cambridge, MA: MIT Press.

McKay, M., M. Davis, and P. Fanning. 1995. *Messages: The Communication Skills Book*. Oakland, CA: New Harbinger Publications.

Monroe, S., and A. D. Simons. 1991. Diathesis-stress theories in the context of life stress research: Implications for the depressive disorders. *Psychological Bulletin* 110:406-425.

Mueser, K. T. 1998. Social skills training and problem solving. in A. S. Bellack and M. Hersen (Eds.) *Comprehensive Clinical Psychology (Volume 6)*, pp. 183-201. New York: Elsevier.

Murphy, P. E., J. W. Ciarrocchi, R. L. Piedmont, S. Cheston, M. Peyrot, and G. Fitchett. 2000. The relation of religious belief and practices, depression, and hopelessness in persons with clinical depression. *Journal of Consulting and Clinical Psychology* 68:1102-1106.

Nezu, A. M. 1987. A problem-solving formulation of depression: A literature review and proposal of a pluralistic model. *Clinical Psychology Review* 7:121-144.

Nolen-Hoeksema, S. 2000. The role of rumination in depressive disorders and mixed anxiety/depressive symptoms. *Journal of Abnormal Psychology* 109:504-511.

Paterson, R. 2000. *The Assertiveness Workbook: How to Express Your Ideas and Stand Up for Yourself at Work and in Relationships.* Oakland, CA: New Harbinger Publications.

Prochaska, J. O., and C. C. DiClemente. 1982. Transtheoretical therapy: Toward a more integrative model of change. *Psychotherapy: Theory, Research and Practice* 19:276-288.

Rehm, L. P., A. L. Wagner, and C. Ivens-Tyndal. 2001. Mood disorders: Unipolar and bipolar. In *Comprehensive Handbook of Psychopathology.* Edited by H. E. Adams and P. B. Sutker. New York: Kluwer/Plenum.

Rowa, K., P. J. Bieling, and Z. V. Segal. Forthcoming. Improving outcomes in cognitive behavioral treatment of depression. In *Improving Outcomes and Preventing Relapse Following Cognitive Behavior Therapy: A Clinical Handbook.* Edited by M. M. Antony, D. A. Roth, and R. G. Heimberg. New York: Guilford Press.

Segal, Z. V., J. M. G. Williams, and J. D. Teasdale. 2002. *Mindfulness based cognitive therapy for depression: A new approach to preventing relapse.* New York: Guilford Press.

Segrin, C. 2001. *Interpersonal Processes in Psychological Problems.* New York: Guilford Press.

Selye, H. 1978. *The Stress of Life.* New York: McGraw-Hill.

Sender, P. M. J., V. M. Vernet, L. S. Perez, C. M. Faro, B. M. Rojas, and G. L. Pallisa. 2004. Functional thyroid pathology in the elderly. *Aten Primaria* 34(4):192-197.

Sintzel, F., M. Mallaret, and T. Bougerol. 2004. Potentializing of tricyclics and serotoninergics by thyroid hormones in resistant depressive disorders. *Encephale* 30(3):267-275.

Stangl, G. I., F. J. Schwarz, and M. Kirchgessner. 1999. Cobalt deficiency effects on trace elements, hormones and enzymes involved in energy metabolism of cattle. *International Journal for Vitamin and Nutrition Research* 69:120-126.

Surks, M. I., and E. Ocampo. 1996. Subclinical thyroid disease. *American Journal of Medicine* 100:217-223.

Tannen, D. 1991. *That's Not What I Meant: How Conversational Style Makes or Breaks Relationships.* New York: Ballantine Books.

Tannen, D. 2001. *You Just Don't Understand: Women and Men in Conversation.* New York: Quill.

Tkachuk, G. A., and G. L. Martin. 1999. Exercise therapy for patients with psychiatric disorders: Research and clinical implications. *Professional Psychology: Research and Practice* 30:275-282.

Ware, J. C., and C. M. Morin. 1997. Sleep in depression and anxiety. In *Understanding Sleep: The Evaluation and Treatment of Sleep Disorders.* Edited by M. R. Pressman and W. C. Orr. Washington, DC: American Psychological Association.

Weissman, M. M. 2000. *Mastering Depression Through Interpersonal Psychotherapy: Patient Workbook.* San Antonio, TX: Psychological Corporation.

Wiersinga, W. M. 1995. Subclinical hypothyroidism and hyperthyroidism: I. Prevalence and clinical relevance. *Netherlands Journal of Medicine* 46:197-204.

Wilson, E. D. 1991. *Wilson's Syndrome: The Miracle of Feeling Well.* Orlando, FL: Cornerstone Publishing.

Winsa, B., H. O. Adami, R. Bergstrom, A. Gamstedt, P. A. Dahlberg, U. Adamson, et al. 1991. Stressful life events and Graves' disease. *Lancet* 338:1475-1479.

Wright, S. A. 2002. Iodine deficiency in the US. *Boston Globe* (July 22, 2002), p.A-3.

Gary S. Ross, MD, is in private practice, specializing in the treatment of thyroid conditions. His focus is a holistic approach that allows the suffering patient to overcome both the physical and psychological symptoms.

Peter J. Bieling, Ph.D., is the manager for the Mood, Anxiety, and Women's Health Concerns Clinic at St. Joseph's Hospital and assistant professor in the department of psychiatry at McMaster's University. He is a specialist in using CBT to treat depression.

Some Other
New Harbinger Titles

The Cyclothymia Workbook, Item 383X, $18.95

The Matrix Repatterning Program for Pain Relief, Item 3910, $18.95

Transforming Stress, Item 397X, $10.95

Eating Mindfully, Item 3503, $13.95

Living with RSDS, Item 3554 $16.95

The Ten Hidden Barriers to Weight Loss, Item 3244 $11.95

The Sjogren's Syndrome Survival Guide, Item 3562 $15.95

Stop Feeling Tired, Item 3139 $14.95

Responsible Drinking, Item 2949 $18.95

The Mitral Valve Prolapse/Dysautonomia Survival Guide,
Item 3031 $14.95

Stop Worrying Abour Your Health, Item 285X $14.95

The Vulvodynia Survival Guide, Item 2914 $15.95

The Multifidus Back Pain Solution, Item 2787 $12.95

Move Your Body, Tone Your Mood, Item 2752 $17.95

The Chronic Illness Workbook, Item 2647 $16.95

Coping with Crohn's Disease, Item 2655 $15.95

The Woman's Book of Sleep, Item 2493 $14.95

The Trigger Point Therapy Workbook, Item 2507 $19.95

Fibromyalgia and Chronic Myofascial Pain Syndrome, second edition,
Item 2388 $19.95

Kill the Craving, Item 237X $18.95

Rosacea, Item 2248 $13.95

Thinking Pregnant, Item 2302 $13.95

Call **toll free, 1-800-748-6273,** or log on to our online bookstore at **www.newharbinger.com** to order. Have your Visa or Mastercard number ready. Or send a check for the titles you want to New Harbinger Publications, Inc., 5674 Shattuck Ave., Oakland, CA 94609. Include $4.50 for the first book and 75¢ for each additional book, to cover shipping and handling. (California residents please include appropriate sales tax.) Allow two to five weeks for delivery.

Prices subject to change without notice.